I0103445

Nordic walking, urban poling, poling or pole walking?

Don't let the terminology confuse you—the above names are all interchangeable, and their purpose, technique and benefits are all the same. Urban poling, a contemporary version of traditional European Nordic walking, uses super-safe grab-and-go strapless ergonomic handles.

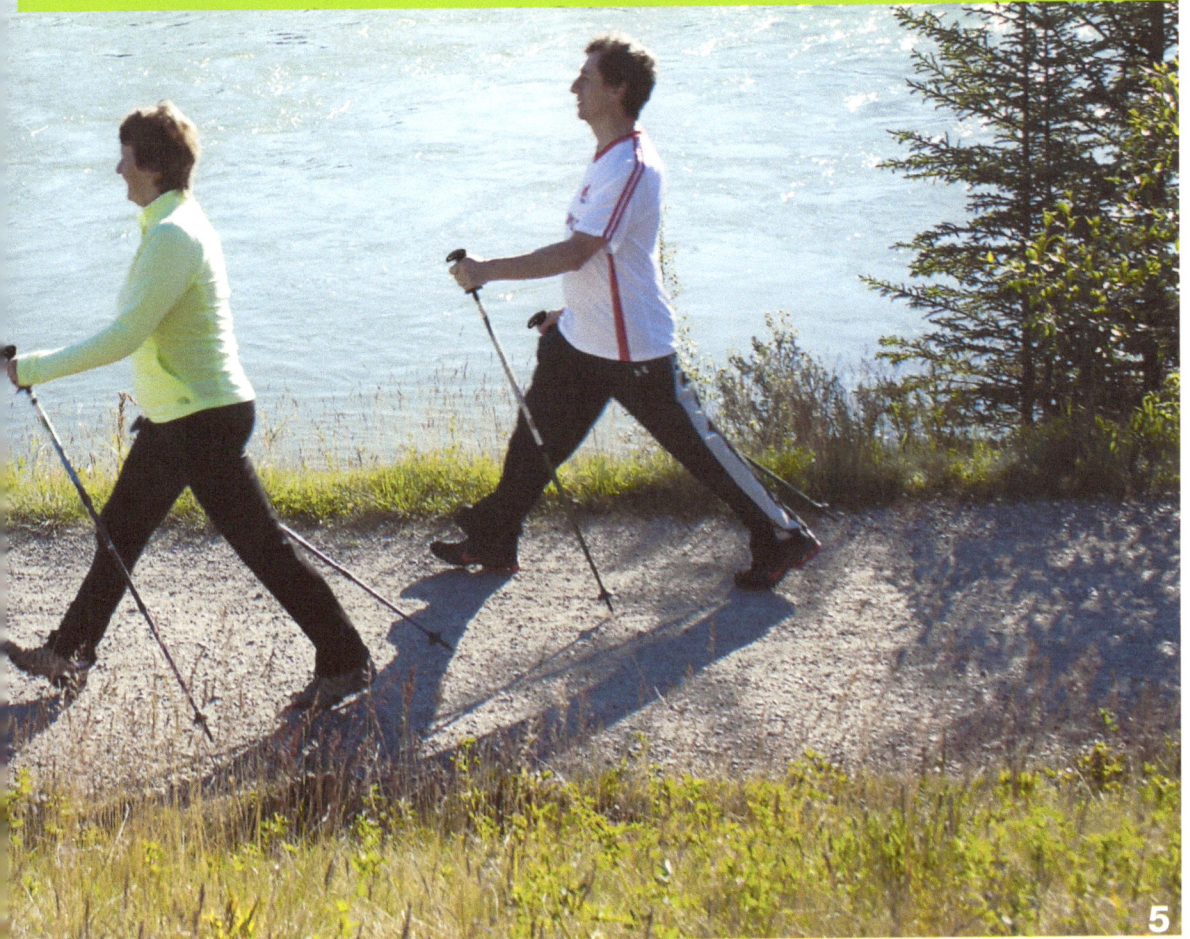

What's All the Excitement?

Over 10 million people call themselves regular Nordic walkers. Here's why.

1. Improves slouchy posture by targeting your upper back muscles.

2. Strengthens and tones your core and upper body.

3. Helps with balance and stability.

4. Unloads weight from your spine and lower body joints.

5. Burns up to 46 percent more calories than standard walking.

6. The intimidation level is virtually nil.

7. No fancy workout wear required.

8. Exercising in nature is a brilliant mood and health booster. Research repeatedly shows that it lowers blood pressure, worry and stress while simultaneously bumping up feelings of confidence and self-esteem.

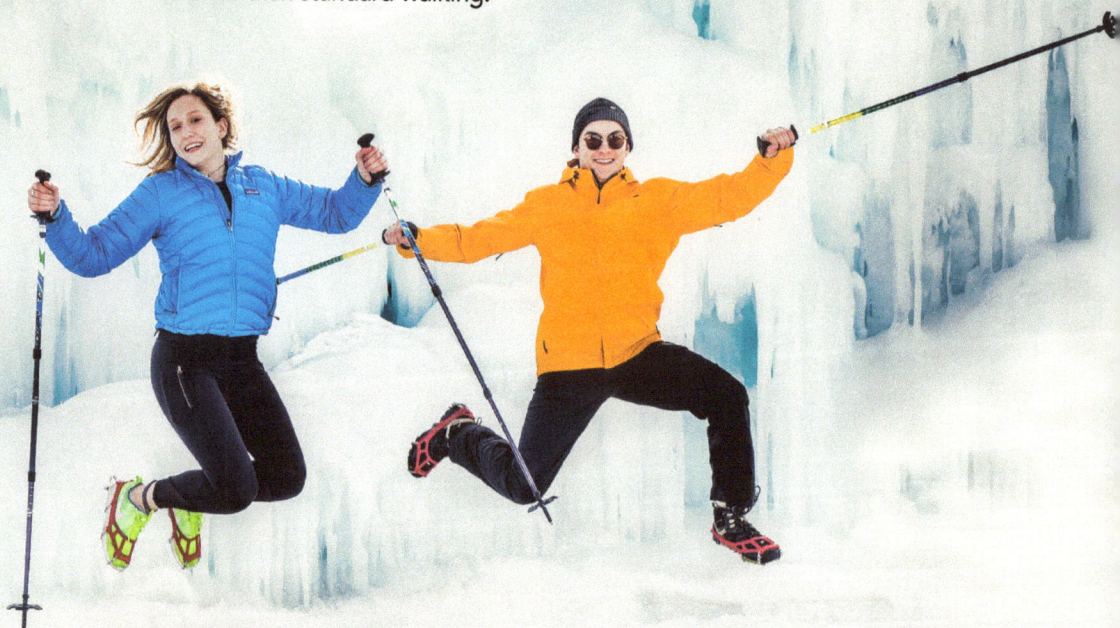

Attention Research Nerds!

Visit www.urbanpoling.com to access 50+ Nordic walking research studies.

Table of Contents

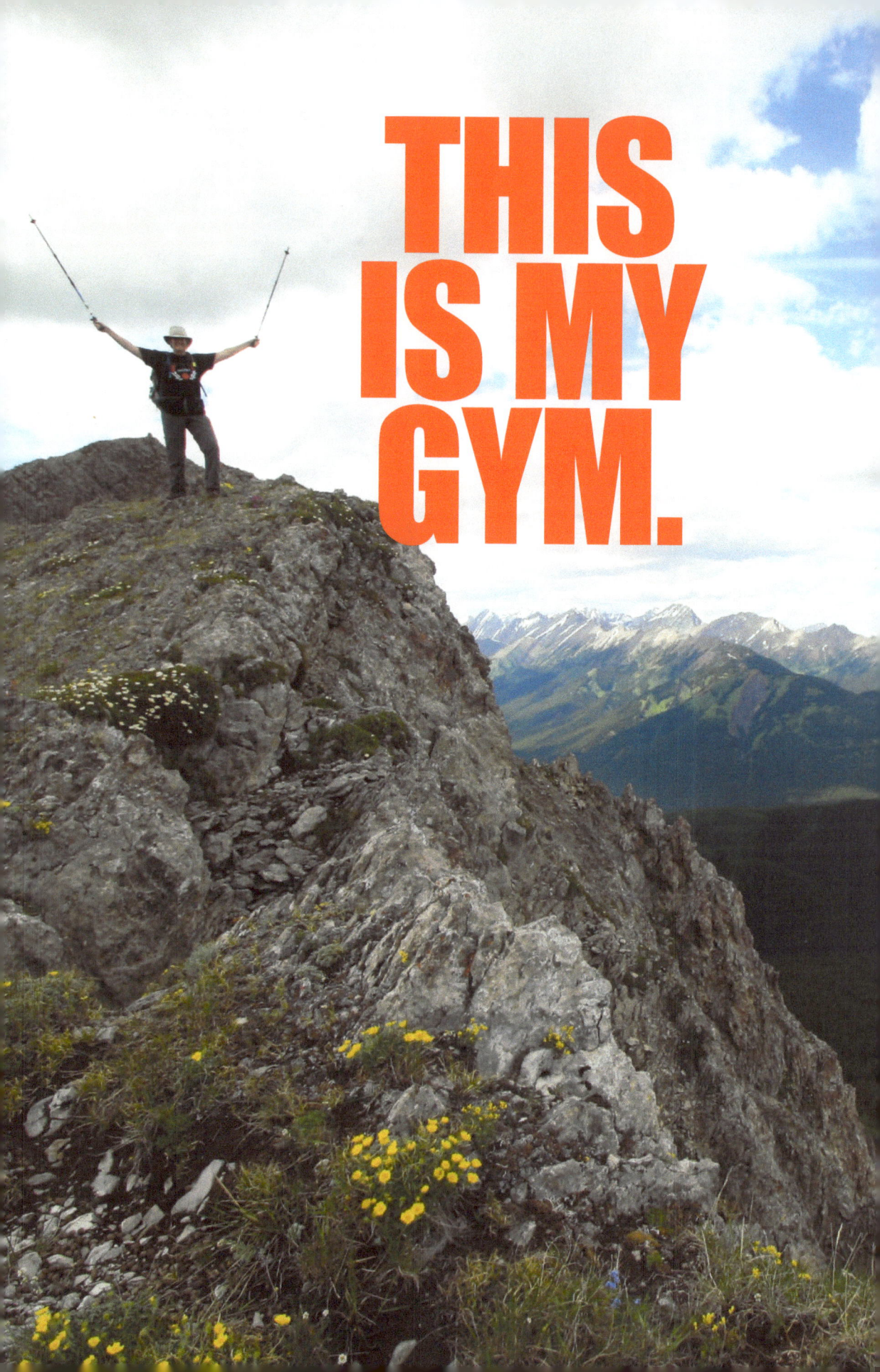

THIS
IS MY
GYM.

FORWARD

A passion for wellness for people of all ages and abilities is what motivated us to design what we believe are the best Nordic walking poles and training programs worldwide.

It all started in Vancouver in 2004 when Mandy's Swedish neighbour took her for her first Nordic walk. An almost immediate "ah-ha" moment–followed up with a dive into the overwhelmingly positive research on the activity–led to the formation of Urban Poling Inc.

Today, we're proud to be Canada's leading Nordic walking pole manufacturer and distributor and to have trained and certified over 5,000 instructors and rehabilitation therapists. The enthusiasm for Nordic walking keeps growing as we expand internationally.

As enthusiastic Nordic walkers and hikers, we are fortunate to do what we love for a living. We are excited to introduce this book and its loads of helpful advice to help you to enjoy Nordic walking in all seasons and for life!

One quick reminder: If you have a chronic health condition, be sure to get your healthcare professional's approval before starting this or any new activity program.

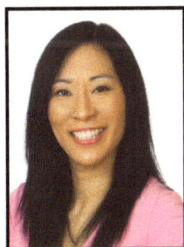

Mandy Shintani
co-director
Urban Poling Inc.

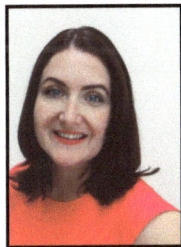

Diana Oliver
co-director
Urban Poling Inc.

INTRODUCTION

If you're reading this book you've likely just bought Nordic walking poles–but now you're stumped and not quite sure how to get started. Or perhaps you're already hooked on Nordic walking and are anxious for more information. Or maybe you're just curious about Nordic walking because you've heard so much about it from friends or in the news.

Barb Gormley
author, director of education & master trainer, Urban Poling Inc.

Whether you've just unclipped your poles for the first time or you're a seasoned pro, this guide is for you.

While the technique isn't difficult, contrary to popular belief, Nordic walking technique isn't intuitive. To experience all the benefits it takes some time, tips and a bit of patience.

But once you catch the rhythm, arm swing and coordination, trust me, you'll never look back!

This book has three objectives:

1. To familiarize you with your Nordic walking poles and to teach you proper Nordic walking technique.
2. To familiarize you with your ACTIVATOR walking poles and to teach you proper ACTIVATOR walking technique.
3. To share loads of inspiring tips and tricks to help you get the very most from your walking pole workouts.

So flip the page, and let's get started!

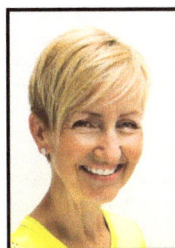

Want to get in touch?
Have a story or suggestion to share? I'd love to hear from you. Connect with me at **barb@urbanpoling.com, www.urbanpoling.com** or **www.BarbGormley.com**.

Nordic Walking: A Quick History

It's always good to know a bit of the back story when you take on a new activity.

1960s/1970s

A Finnish physical education teacher introduces walking with ski poles to her students. Later, a Finnish cross-country skiing coach promotes a similar activity for competitive athletes and advanced exercisers.

1980s

Europeans begin showing interest in the benefits of adding modified poles to standard walking. Late in the decade, an American entrepreneur introduces a strapless walking pole with angled rubber boot tips.

1990s

A Finnish ski pole manufacturer introduces a walking pole, also with angled rubber boot tips, and coins the term "Nordic walking."

2000s

Nordic walking begins spreading worldwide, and more companies begin manufacturing Nordic walking poles. Nordic walking associations and instructor certification programs appear in several countries.

Urban Poling Inc., currently Canada's largest Nordic walking pole manufacturer and distributer, is established in 2005. Over 10 years, it introduces five editions of poles as well as instructor certification programs.

TODAY

Over 10 million people in Norway, Sweden, Finland, Demark, Switzerland, Germany, etc., are regular Nordic walkers. Every year Nordic walking grows in popularity in countries such as Canada, the U.K. and the U.S.

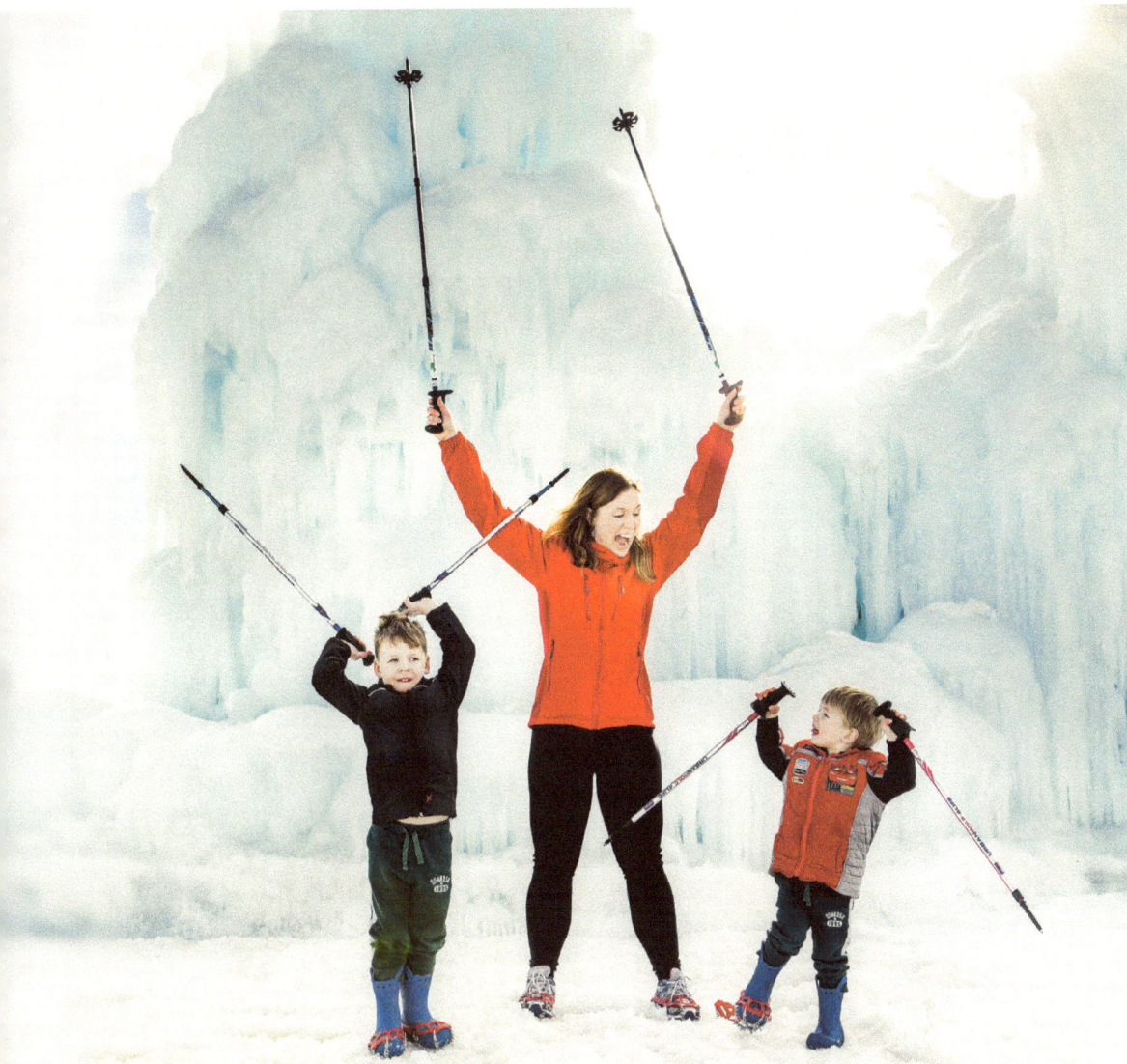

9. Increases your shoulders' range of motion and muscular endurance, which is especially important after breast cancer surgery.

10. Challenges your non-dominant (weaker) arm to match the strength and coordination of your dominant (stronger) arm.

11. Nordic walking's level of perceived exertion is similar to standard walking, even though it helps burn more calories and involves more muscles.

12. Similar to swimming, tennis and bowling, you can continue Nordic walking into your later years. The technique is exactly the same for everyone, but your pace may slow as you age.

13. You'll likely have the same poles for a lifetime. Only the boot tips need to be replaced approximately every six to 12 months.

14. There are numerous Nordic walking instructor-led classes and casual groups where you can walk and socialize with others.

15. Physicians, physiotherapists, occupational therapists and other health care professionals regularly recommend Nordic walking as an effective, safe and enjoyable way to improve your health.

Get to Know Your Nordic Walking Poles

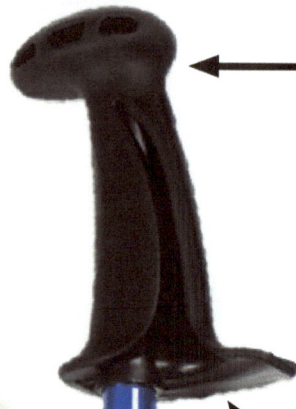

COREGRIP HANDLE

Thick ergonomic handles absorb vibrations and prevent grip fatigue during long walks. No fumbling with straps when you reach for your water bottle or sunscreen

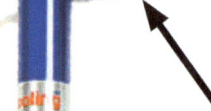

LEDGE

Press onto the Ledge to feel your core muscles, back of your arms and sides of your trunk tighten and propel your body forward.

UPPER SECTION

TREKKING BASKETS & SNOW BASKETS

(Adventure poles only or purchase separately) Trekking baskets keep the carbide tips from sinking into mud or between rocks. Snow baskets keep your poles from disappearing into deep snow while snowshoeing.

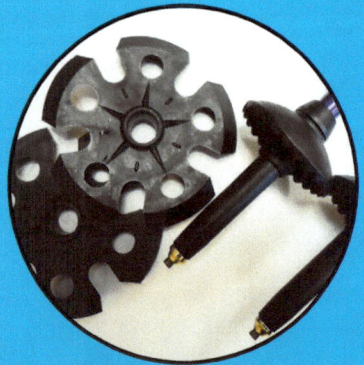

URBANPOLE 300

FERRULE

Dampens vibrations and connects the upper and lower sections of your poles. It doesn't turn, so don't touch it!

LOWER SECTION

ALL ABOUT BOOT TIPS

1. Turn them so the toes are pointing back behind you.
2. Push and pull them on and off (no need to twist).
3. Check the treads regularly. Worn treads don't grip the ground or absorb shock well.
4. The life of your boot tips depends on the frequency and distance of your walks, the roughness of the walking surfaces, and how frequently you drag (versus lift and lower) them. Replace them about every 6–12 months.

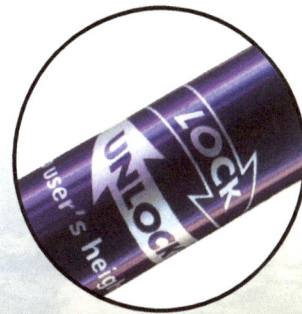

LOCK/UNLOCK

Check here to tighten or loosen your poles. (Remember: turn the upper and lower sections of the poles not the ferrule).

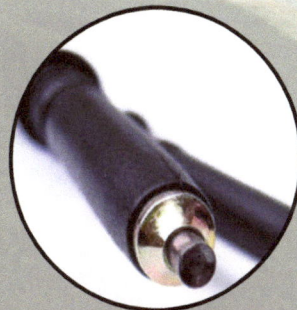

BOOT TIP

Provides a springy yet solid landing for each pole plant.

CARBIDE TIP

Ideal for grass, sand, trails and other soft surfaces.

How to Set Up Your Nordic Walking Poles

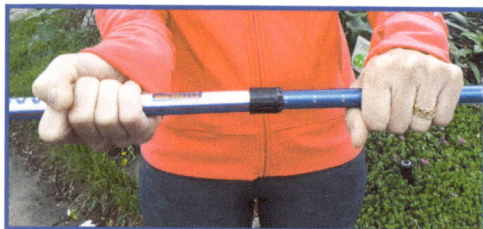

STEP 1

Place one hand on the lower section and one hand on the upper section. Turn the lower section three or four turns in the direction of the "unlock" arrow. Pull out the bottom section to lengthen the pole.

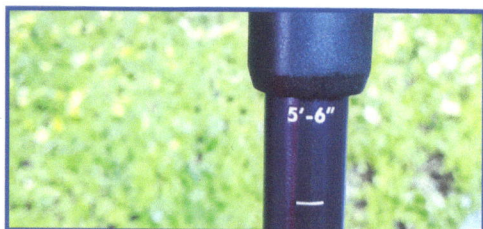

STEP 2

Look for your height marked on the lower section of the pole (centimetres are on one side and inches on the other side).

Tip: When you're a beginner, set the poles to your height minus two inches to make them more manageable. For example, if you're 5'8", set your poles at 5'6". (Try them at your full height once you have some Nordic walking experience.)

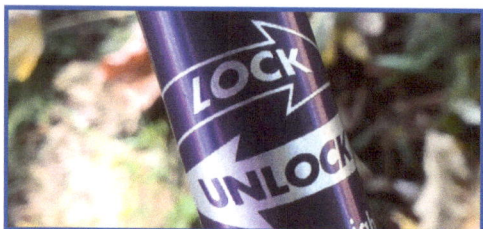

STEP 3

Lock the pole firmly in place by turning the lower section several turns in the direction of the "lock" arrow. Don't try to turn the fixed black plastic ferrule! Hold above and below it.

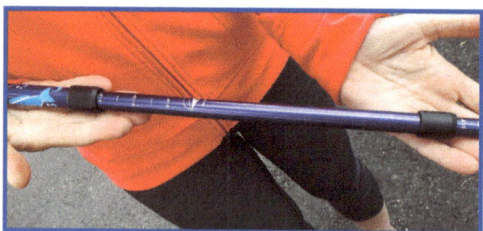

Important: Urban Poling Adventure poles are three-section (versus two-section) poles and, therefore, they have two ferrules. To lengthen these poles, follow the above instructions and then repeat the process a second time lengthening the pole at the second ferrule.

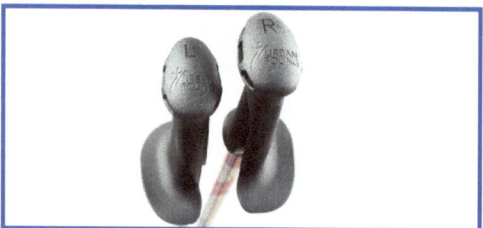

STEP 4

Hold the poles so the R and L on the top of the handles are in the appropriate hands. Adjust the boot tips so they point back behind you.

HELP! MY POLES ARE STUCK

5 quick ways to release a stuck pole:

1 Be sure you're turning the lower section of the pole in the direction of the "unlock" arrow.

2 The buddy system: have a friend hold one end of the pole with two hands while you turn the other end with two hands.

3 Wear rubber gloves for a better grip.

4 Invert the pole, secure the handle between your feet and then turn with both hands.

5 Place the pole outside in the winter air or in a freezer, or apply cold packs to the lower section of the pole. The metal components will contract faster than the plastic ferrule and will loosen the connection.

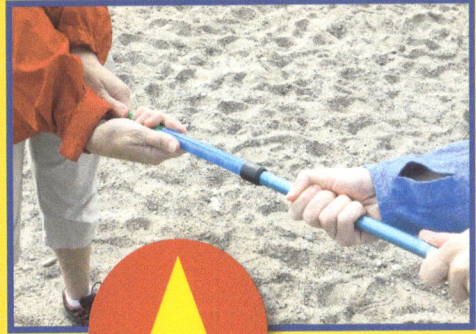

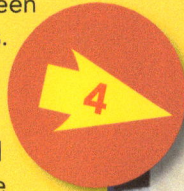

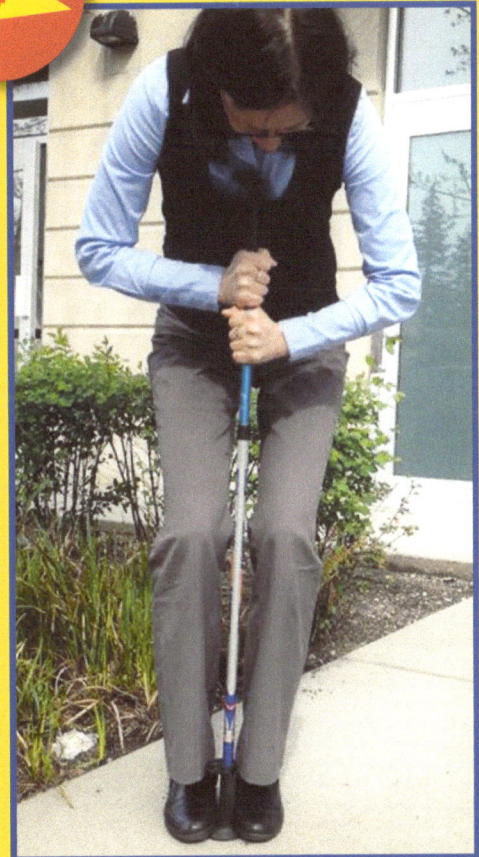

More Equipment Tips

1 Never lock your poles beyond the words "Stop" (printed on the very end of the lower section of each pole).

2 In extremely cold weather, poles that have been stored indoors may gradually shorten after a few minutes of walking (as the metal lower section contracts but the plastic ferrule retains its size). To resolve this issue, place your poles outdoors for a few minutes before you adjust their length. Or stop and check your poles after a few minutes of walking to ensure they have retained their length. Or once your poles have been used in cold weather, simply always leave them at their extended length.

3 With just a bit of practice you will be able to lengthen and shorten your poles with ease. Never use tools or lubricants of any kind on any part of your poles.

11

How to Nordic Walk

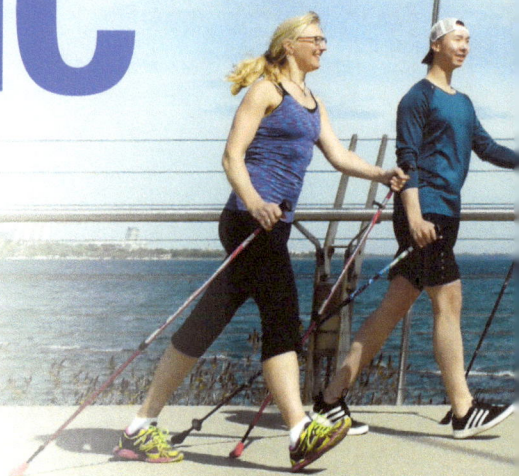

BEFORE YOU START MOVING:

- Without your poles, take a brisk walk of 20–30 steps. Notice how your arms naturally swing like long pendulums from the shoulders (not the elbows) and how your opposite arm and leg move together. Don't over-think this—just walk normally. Remember this natural gait as you begin Step 1.

- Pull your navel up and in, lift your ribcage and relax your shoulders. This posture tightens your abs, lengthens your spine, prevents your hips from shifting side to side as you walk, and helps you control your poles.

- Hold your poles with an easy grip—not too tight and not too loose.

PLAN FOR BREAKS

When you lose your rhythm or feel frustrated, stop to regroup. Roll your shoulders back a few times to relax them, take some deep breaths and do a favourite stretch. Then start Nordic walking again refreshed.

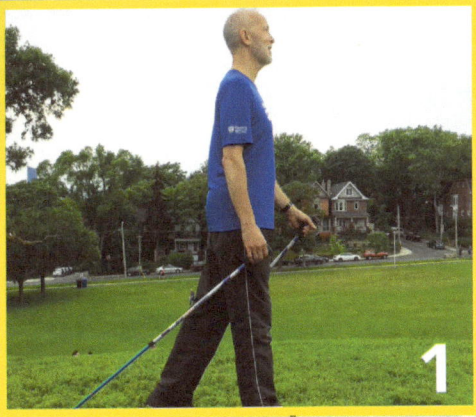

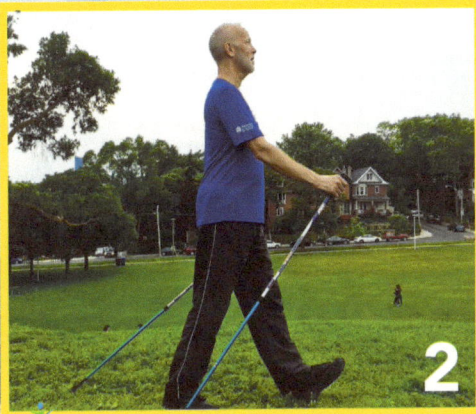

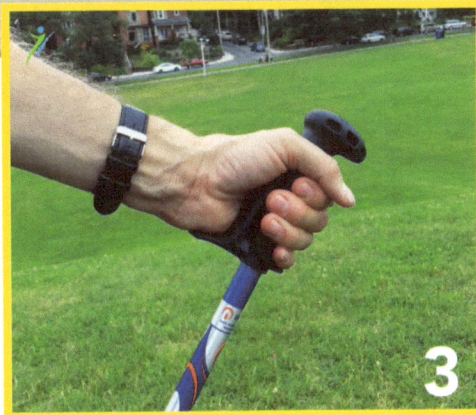

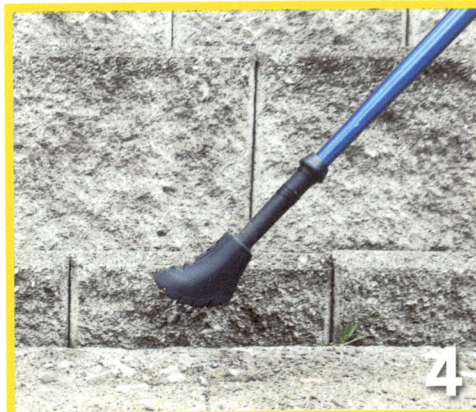

STEP 1 WALK AND DRAG YOUR POLES

Holding your poles, stand with your arms straight and your thumbs beside your thighs so your boot tips are on the ground and well behind you. Begin walking, dragging your poles behind you. Be sure that your opposite arm and leg move together.

TIP: As you walk, relax and pretend your poles aren't there.

STEP 2 STEP A LITTLE LONGER, SWING A LITTLE HIGHER

Continue walking, but make your steps a little longer and swing your arms up a little higher to a handshake-height position. Keep your arms swinging like long pendulums. Let your thumbs return back beside your thighs with each swing.

TIP: You've swung high enough in front if you feel your boot tips catching on the ground behind you.

STEP 3 PRESS AND PROPEL

Begin pressing the outside edges of your hands onto the Ledge of the handles each time a boot tip lands.

TIP: Continue pushing your thumbs right down to the sides of your thighs. Feel your abs and the back of your arms and shoulders contracting and your poles propelling you forward.

STEP 4 ADD A LITTLE LIFT

Instead of dragging your boot tips, begin to lift them (just a centimetre or so off the ground) and firmly plant them.

TA DA! Once you can coordinate all four of these steps, you're officially Nordic walking with great style. 🏃 *and technique.*

Nordic Walking Warm-Up

A warm-up isn't always required for Nordic walking, but starting out with some simple movements performed with an easy energy always feels good. Create your own warm-up by choosing 3 or 4 of the following exercises.

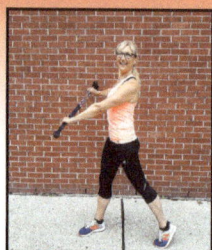
waist rotations

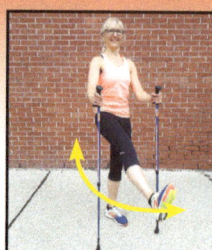
leg swings

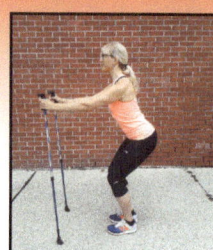
mini squats

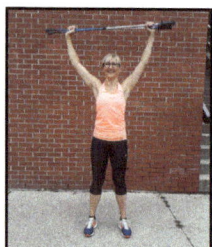
overhead reaches

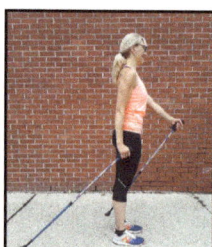
alternating arm swings

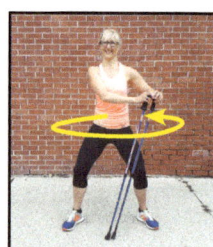
stir the pot

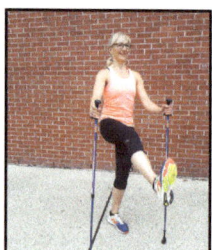
ankle circles

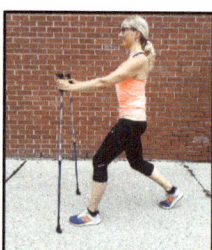
mini lunges

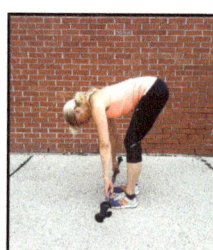
roll down & up

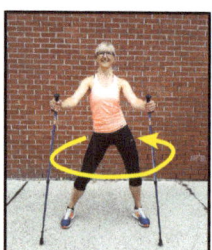
hoolahoop

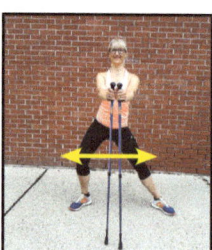
mini side lunges

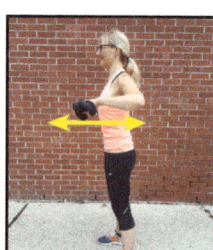
rows

40 Minute Full-Body Workout

Add a little variety to your walks with stationary exercise intervals. Modify the exercises as required.

START > WARM UP

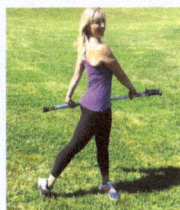
waist rotations

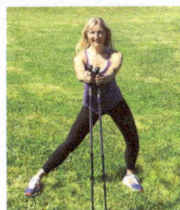
side lunges

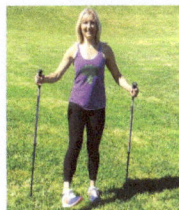
ankle rotations

30 sec. each ▼

UPPER BODY & CORE CONDITIONING

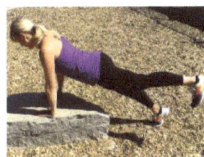
plank with alternating leg lift

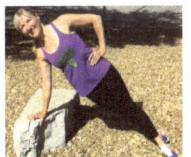
static side plank

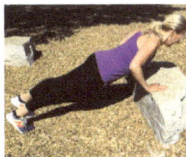
push ups

30 sec. each ▼

NORDIC WALK

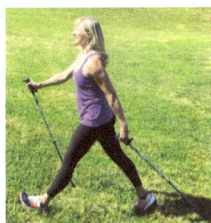

16 mins ▼

UPPER BODY & CORE CONDITIONING

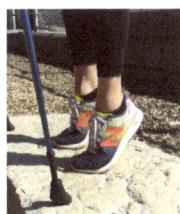
calf raises

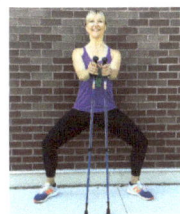
jumping jacks

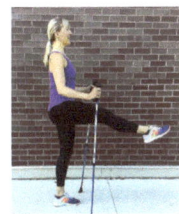
alternating front kicks

30 sec. each ▼

NORDIC WALK

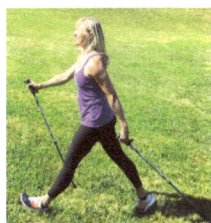

16 mins ▼

FINISH > STRETCH & COOLDOWN

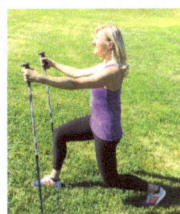
hip flexors

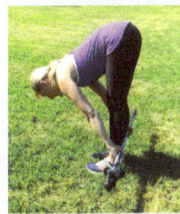
hamstrings

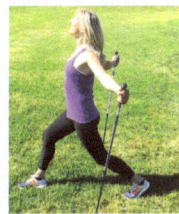
chest & shoulders

Hold 30 sec. and perform each **twice**

WHAT (NOT) TO WEAR

Hat and sunglasses? Check. Sunscreen? Check. Here are a few additional suggestions to help keep you warm in the cold and cool in the heat.

WEAR THIS	WHY IT'S BETTER	NOT THAT
Tights, shorts or non-baggy pants	Streamlined clothing is more comfortable for physical activity. Look for fabric with stretch.	Big loose sweat pants or tight confining pants
Hiking-style shorts	Hiking shorts have multiple pockets for stashing your boot tips, tissues, phone and other small items.	Yoga or workout shorts
Wind pants (as a top layer), fleece-lined pants or ski pants	While fine in warm dry weather, jeans absorb moisture from rain and snow and are not windproof.	Jeans
Waist- or thigh-length jacket	A long coat can impede your stride. Avoid super-puffy coats that can slow down your arm action.	Below-the-knee jacket
Layers of tight thin tops	Bulky clothing can prevent your arms from swinging easily. Multiple thin layers retain more heat in cold weather.	One or two baggy or bulky tops
Perspiration-wicking fabrics, fleece and down	Cotton retains moisture and can create chaffing and blisters. High-tech fabrics, fleece and down are lightweight and warm, and they dry quickly.	Cotton clothing and socks
Sports bra	A sports bra retains its fit when wet.	Lingerie bra
Buff (a seamless tube of stretchy fabric that can be worn as a scarf, headband, cap, wristband or face mask)	Unlike a bulky scarf, a buff can be tucked into a pocket once you're warm and no longer need it.	Long scarf
Light supportive running shoes, trail shoes or hiking shoes/boots	Dry and comfortable feet make a workout more enjoyable and help prevent blisters.	Casual sandals or worn-out running shoes
Warm, flexible and windproof mittens or gloves	Choose an option that blocks the wind and keeps your fingers warm but that also allows you to feel the ledge of your poles.	Very bulky or stiff gloves or mittens; knit mittens; light running gloves

Do It Right!

Don't miss out on any of the strength, posture and conditioning benefits of Nordic walking. Use these technique tips to check and perfect your form.

1 LOOK

Keeping your eyes focused forward, not down, initiates a positive chain reaction: eyes up, head up, shoulders back and chest lifted.

2 RELAX

Pressing your shoulders down avoids unnecessary tension across the top of your shoulders. Keeping your shoulder joints loose lets your arms swing freely.

3 EXTEND

Swinging your arms like long pendulums (not like a choo-choo train) keeps the weight of the poles away from your core requiring it to tighten with each forward swing.

4 PRESS

Exerting a downward pressure on the Ledge and holding the handles with an easy grip creates a bracing effect in the core.

5 LIFT

Pulling your navel up and in helps to brace your core creating a stable foundation for your swinging arms.

6 LENGTHEN

Striding just a little longer than when standard walking energizes your walk and encourages your arms to stay long.

7 PLANT

Landing the opposite boot tip and foot simultaneously, creating one firm boot tip/foot landing sound, ensures a constant and stable base of support.

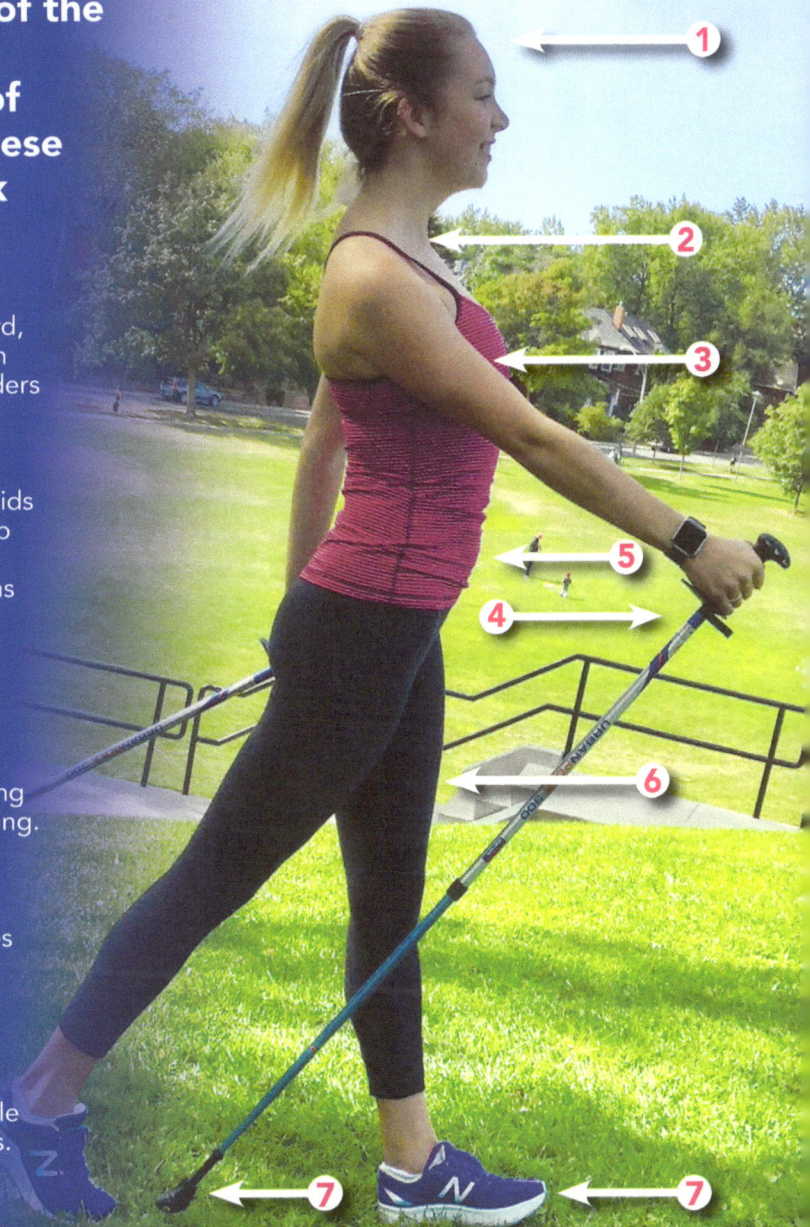

HOW FIT ARE YOU?

Assess your starting point then track your progress with this simple 3-minute fitness test

Here's some great news: researchers around the world report that regular Nordic walking can help improve your muscular strength, endurance, flexibility and balance.

In fact, when compared to standard walking, Nordic walking wins by leaps and bounds.

In one study, subjects Nordic walked twice a week for 60 minutes for nine weeks. A control group performed the same walking routine but without poles.

After just nine weeks, all participants improved in all categories. However, the Nordic walking group showed dramatically more improvement:

- The Nordic walking group improved 15% in the chair stand, 20% in the arm curl and 14% on the step-in-place (see exercise descriptions on the next page).

- The control group improved 2%, 3% and 4% respectively.

To conduct your own personal research, assess your starting fitness level by performing the same three exercises used in the study. Then Nordic walk for 60 minutes twice a week (modify this however you like, of course) for nine weeks. After nine weeks perform the three exercises again to determine your improvement.

Source: *Improvements in Functional Capacity From Nordic Walking: A Randomized Controlled Trial Among Older Adults*, Parkatti, Perttunen & Wacker, 2012

IMPORTANT! Perform each exercise to the best of your ability, but don't push yourself to a point of overexertion or beyond what you think is safe for you.

#1 CHAIR STAND

Sit with your feet flat on the floor. Stand up, and then sit back down. Repeat for 30 seconds.

# of repetitions: _____

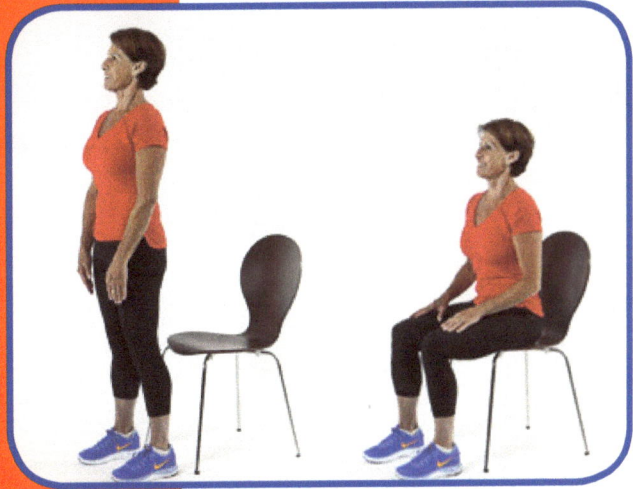

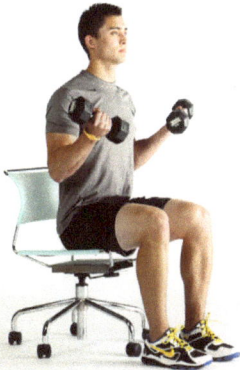

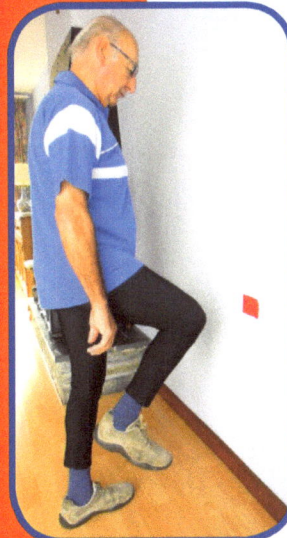

#2 ARM CURL

In a seated position, hold a pair of weights (perhaps 5–8 lb.) with your arms extended at your sides. Curl them toward your shoulders, then lower them to the start position. Repeat for 30 seconds.

# of repetitions: _____

#3 STEP-IN-PLACE

Place a piece of tape on a wall midway between your knees and hips. March in place for two minutes, gently tapping the tape each time. Rest as required; hold the wall or a chair if desired.

# of repetitions: _____

7 THINGS EVERY NEW NORDIC WALKER SHOULD KNOW

Set yourself up for success with this wise advice

1 It takes time
You won't master the technique in the first few minutes of trying it. Most people, including the super-fit and highly-coordinated, need at least two or three (or four or five or more) times to feel competent.

2 You have a strong (and not so strong) side
Your non-dominant arm might not fully cooperate in the beginning. If the boot tip on your weaker side keeps slipping, be sure you are truly swinging all the way up to a handshake position.

3 You'll be tired
Nordic walking uses almost every muscle in your body and burns up to 20 percent more calories than standard walking. Keep your first outings with your poles shorter rather than longer.

4 You'll get sweaty
Dress as if it were 10 degrees warmer than the actual temperature. In the fall and winter you will feel chilly at the start but be just the right temperature within 10 minutes.

5 You're an early adopter
While researchers and millions of fans know that Nordic walking is an almost-perfect exercise activity, not everyone is clued-in. When bystanders look at you quizzically or ask "Where's the snow?," just smile knowingly and keep moving.

6 Winter might throw you off-stride
When winter temperatures or icy sidewalks prevent you from exercising outdoors, have an indoor back-up plan. Some shopping malls offer early morning walking, and some schools, community centres and military bases also open their doors for walkers.

7 Friends are everything
When you're feeling tired, lazy or just too busy, the camaraderie and support of a walking buddy or group can do wonders to keep your Nordic walking workouts on track.

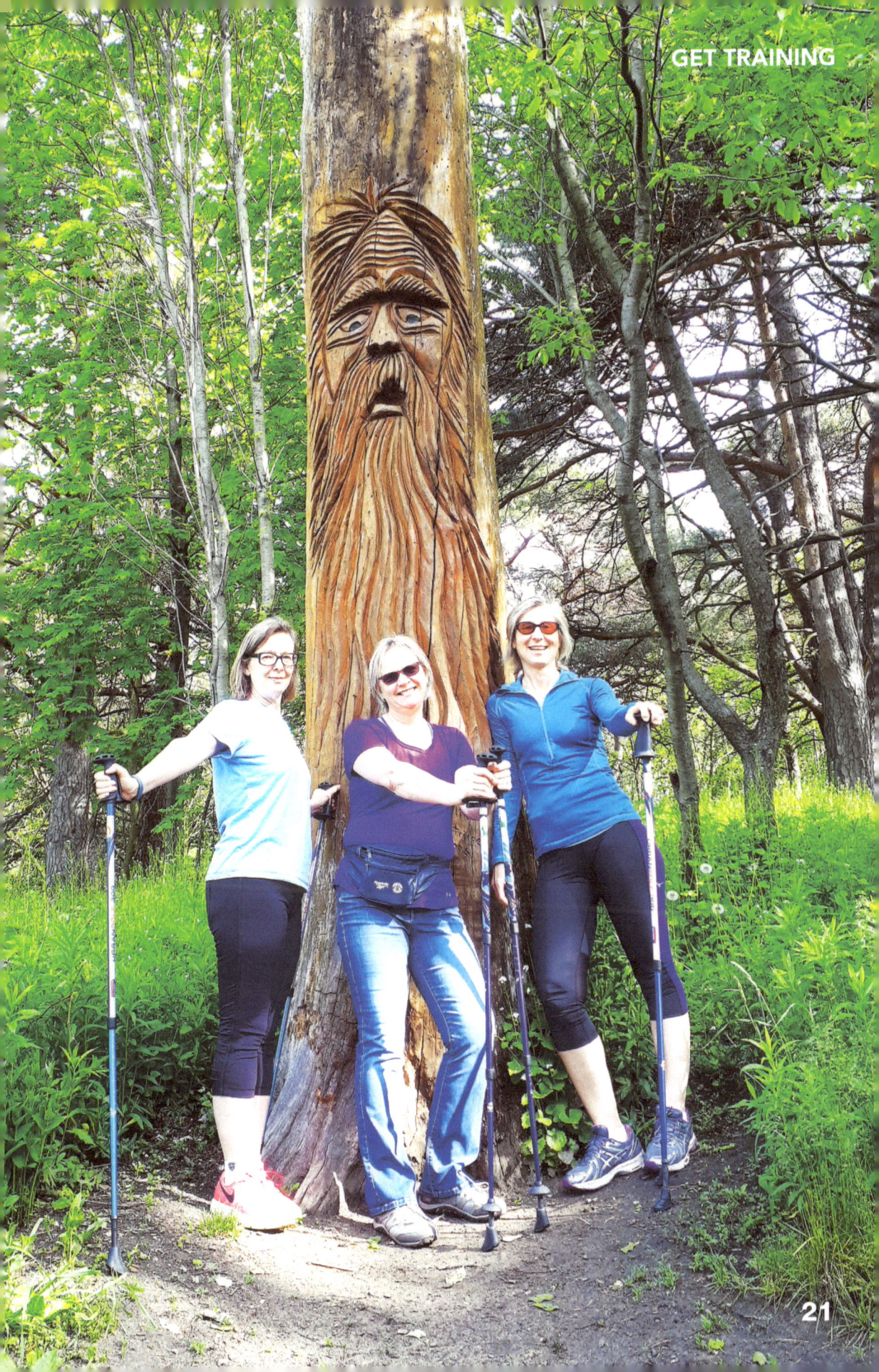

6 WEEKS TO FIT!

Try this BEGINNER'S training program that takes you from standard walking to Nordic walking 5km or more.

WEEK 1	WEEK 2	WEEK 3	WEEK 4	WEEK 5	WEEK 6
MONDAY easy Nordic walk 15-20 min.	**MONDAY** easy Nordic walk 20-30 min.	**MONDAY** Nordic walk 30-40 min.	**MONDAY** Nordic walk 40-50 min.	**MONDAY** Nordic walk 50-60 min.	**MONDAY** Nordic walk 50-75 min.
TUESDAY active rest	**TUESDAY** active rest	**TUESDAY** active rest	**TUESDAY** active rest	**TUESDAY** active rest	**TUESDAY** active rest
WEDNESDAY easy Nordic walk 15-20 min.	**WEDNESDAY** easy Nordic walk 20-30 min.	**WEDNESDAY** Nordic walk 30-40 min.	**WEDNESDAY** Nordic walk 40-50 min.	**WEDNESDAY** Nordic walk 50-60 min.	**WEDNESDAY** Nordic walk 50-75 min.
THURSDAY active rest	**THURSDAY** active rest	**THURSDAY** active rest	**THURSDAY** active rest	**THURSDAY** active rest	**THURSDAY** active rest
FRIDAY easy Nordic walk 15-20 min.	**FRIDAY** easy Nordic walk 20-30 min.	**FRIDAY** Nordic walk 30-40 min.	**FRIDAY** Nordic walk 40-50 min.	**FRIDAY** Nordic walk 50-60 min.	**FRIDAY** Nordic walk 50-75 min.
SATURDAY crosstrain	**SATURDAY** crosstrain	**SATURDAY** crosstrain	**SATURDAY** crosstrain	**SATURDAY** crosstrain	**SATURDAY** crosstrain
SUNDAY active rest	**SUNDAY** active rest	**SUNDAY** active rest	**SUNDAY** active rest	**SUNDAY** active rest	**SUNDAY** active rest

DEFINITIONS
Crosstrain: an activity unlike Nordic walking, such as, Pilates, swimming, cycling or a fitness class
Active rest: physical activities that are non-taxing, such as, walking your dog, gardening, bike riding and doing simple household chores

IMPORTANT
- Warm up for 2-3 minutes (easy leg swings, arm circles, waist rotations, etc.). Cool down with 5-10 minutes of stretching (see page 28).
- If necessary, revise the walking timeframes to suit your personal abilities.

4 WEEKS TO FIT!

If you're an **INTERMEDIATE/ADVANCED** level walker, use this plan to be Nordic walking 5k in just one month

WEEK 1	WEEK 2	WEEK 3	WEEK 4
MONDAY Nordic walk 30-40 min.	**MONDAY** Nordic walk 40-50 min.	**MONDAY** Nordic walk 50-60 min.	**MONDAY** Nordic walk 50-75 min.
TUESDAY active rest	**TUESDAY** active rest	**TUESDAY** active rest	**TUESDAY** active rest
WEDNESDAY Nordic walk 30-40 min.	**WEDNESDAY** Nordic walk 40-50 min.	**WEDNESDAY** Nordic walk 50-60 min.	**WEDNESDAY** Nordic walk 50-75 min.
THURSDAY active rest	**THURSDAY** active rest	**THURSDAY** active rest	**THURSDAY** active rest
FRIDAY Nordic walk 30-40 min.	**FRIDAY** Nordic walk 40-50 min.	**FRIDAY** Nordic walk 50-60 min.	**FRIDAY** Nordic walk 50-75 min.
SATURDAY crosstrain	**SATURDAY** crosstrain	**SATURDAY** crosstrain	**SATURDAY** crosstrain
SUNDAY active rest	**SUNDAY** active rest	**SUNDAY** active rest	**SUNDAY** active rest

DEFINITIONS
Crosstrain: an activity unlike Nordic walking, such as, Pilates, swimming, cycling or a fitness class
Active rest: physical activities that are non-taxing, such as, walking your dog, gardening, bike riding and doing simple household chores

IMPORTANT
- Warm up for 2-3 minutes (easy leg swings, arm circles, waist rotations, etc.). Cool down with 5-10 minutes of stretching (see page 28).
- If necessary, revise the walking time-frames to suit your personal abilities.

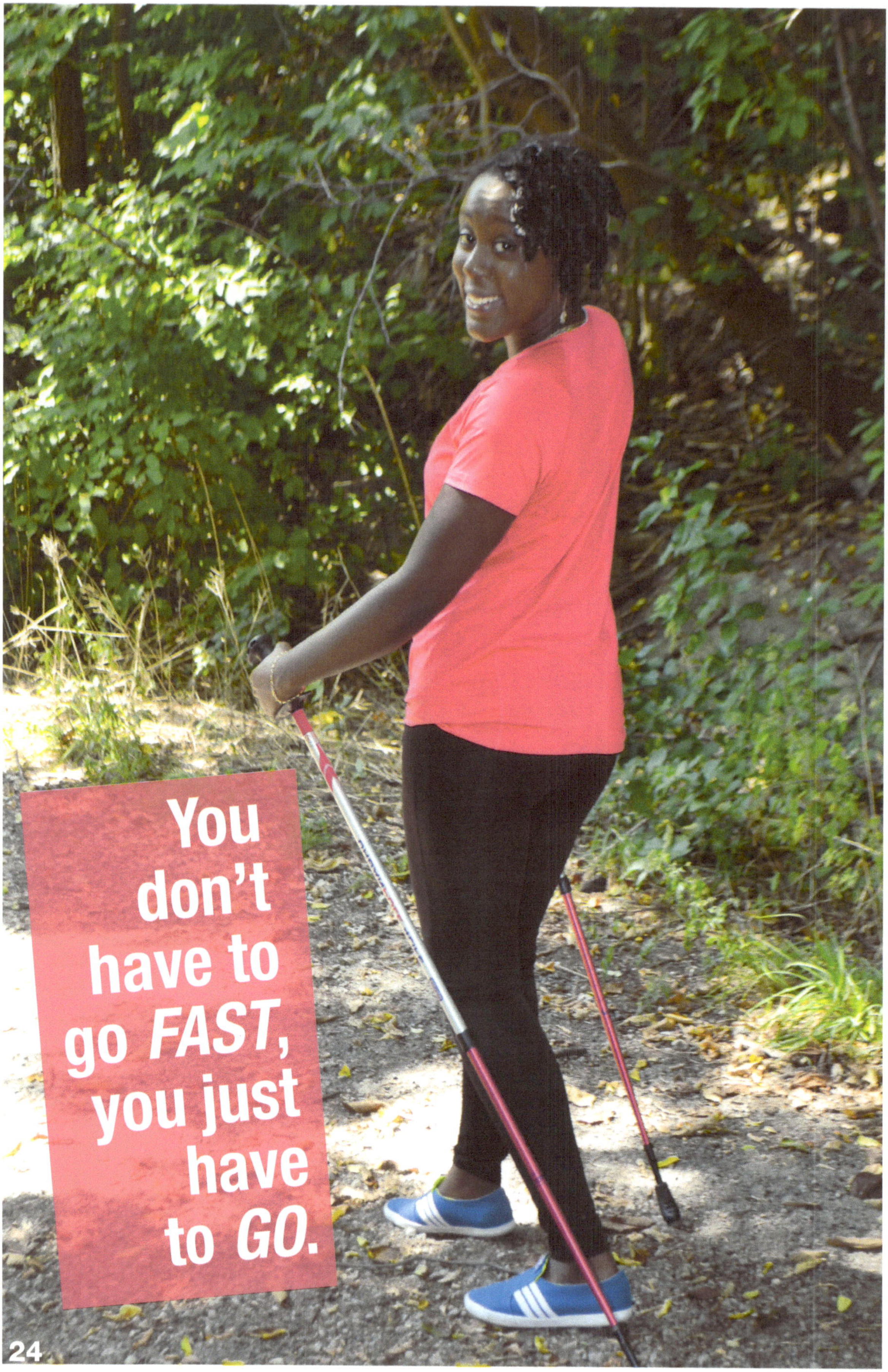
You don't have to go *FAST*, you just have to *GO*.

ROOKIE MISTAKES TO AVOID

BEWARE OF THESE COMMON NORDIC WALKING MISSTEPS.

1. Socializing too much and losing your form

When you're a beginner, even if you're a master multi-tasker, Nordic walking requires a lot of concentration. For your first few Nordic walks, don't assume you'll be able to chat at length with your friends (the way you do when standard walking) and at the same time maintain good technique.

2. Scrimping on shoes

A big box store might be ideal for purchasing laundry soap, biscuits and bulk frozen pizza, but not athletic shoes or boots. Visit a local running/walking shop where a staff member will analyze your gait. (Do you overpronate, supinate or are you neutral?) The right footwear will help keep you injury free, greatly reduce fatigue and take your Nordic walks to a whole new level. Once you've found the perfect shoes replace them regularly, perhaps once a year.

3. Being overly-ambitious

Nordic walking is more physically demanding than standard walking. If you normally walk for 60 minutes without poles, try Nordic walking for about 40 minutes the first few times. Assess how your muscles and energy respond, and then gradually increase the exercise time as you're able.

4. Wearing a bulky backpack

The straps of a backpack, even if the pack isn't heavily loaded, can impede your shoulder movement if you're a beginner. Instead, free up your shoulders by wearing a waist pack or clothing with lots of pockets.

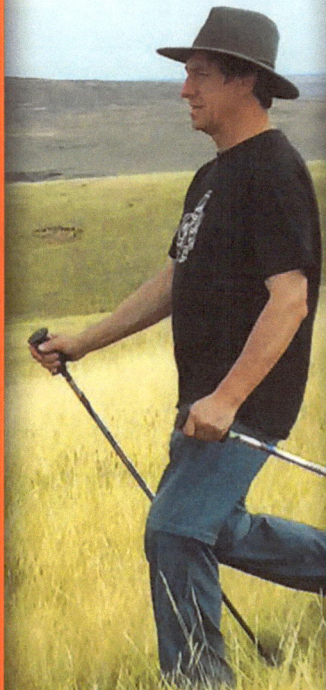

Still prefer a backpack? Go for a higher-end model with a chest strap and ergonomic shoulder straps that curve in towards each other slightly.

5. Overdressing

It is tempting to really bundle up on a cold winter day. But you'll likely be sweaty and steamy after just a few minutes of walking with your poles. Instead, use the runners' rule and dress for weather that is 10 degrees warmer; you'll start out slightly chilly but warm up within a few minutes. Also consider buying clothes designed to help manage heat, for example, a buff (you can store in your pocket when it's no longer needed around your neck) and a jacket with zip-pits (zippered armpits). To help start your walk feeling warm, heat your walking clothes in the drier for a few minutes just before you leave home.

6. Wearing the wrong gloves or mittens

Icy cold hands can ruin an otherwise beautiful walk. When you walk with poles you aren't able to put your hands in your pockets, pull them up into your sleeves or tuck them into your armpits. Mittens with glove liners are usually the warmest. Be sure they're not too bulky; you need to feel the Ledge of your handles.

7. Forgetting sunscreen in strategic areas

The straight-arm technique of Nordic walking fully exposes bare arms and hands to the sun. Remember to apply sunscreen to your arms, the back of your hands, and even the tender skin between your thumb and first finger.

6 MUST-DO STRETCHES
FOR NORDIC WALKERS

Wrap up every walk with this series of feel-good stretches.

1. QUADRICEPS

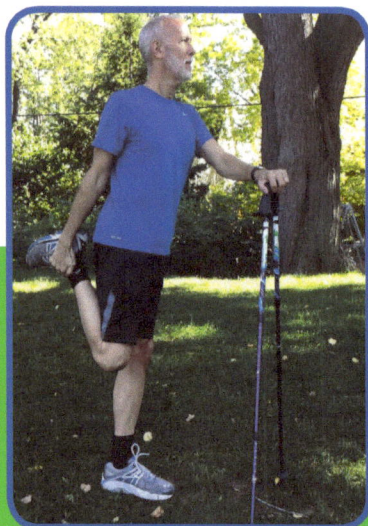

With both poles in one hand for balance, hold one foot with your heel close to your glute. Press your hips forward creating a straight line between your shoulder and knee.

2. HAMSTRINGS

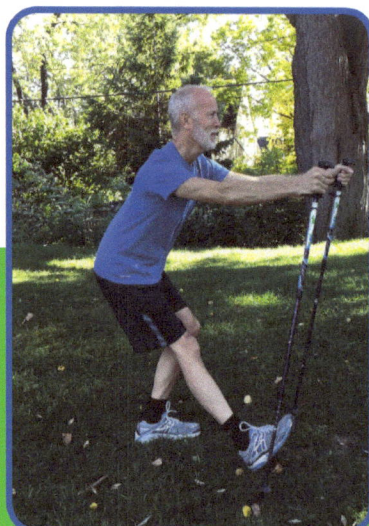

Extend one leg forward bending the standing leg. Hinge forward from the hips, reaching your arms and chest forward.

3. CALVES

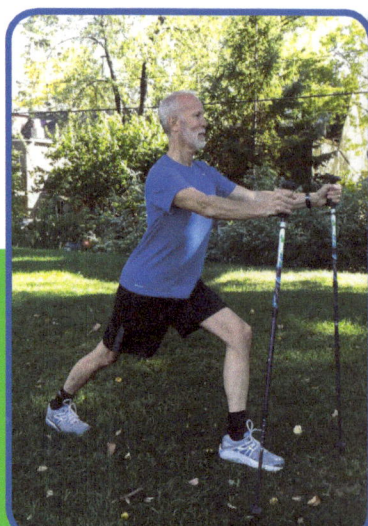

With your poles in front for balance, take a big step back. Align the back heel and toes, bend the front knee and press your back heel down.

Perform each stretch twice per side, holding for 30 seconds each time.

4. CHEST

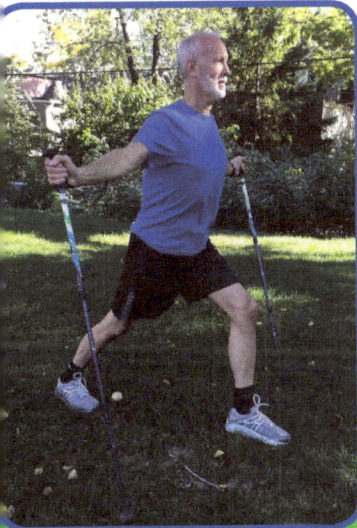

In a lunge position with your poles extended to the side, reach your hands back toward each other and lift your chest and face.

5. SHOULDERS

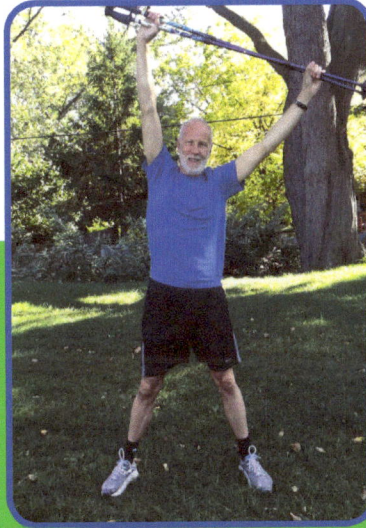

With your feet apart, hold your poles high overhead and press them back gently. Lean slightly to the right and then left to add a gentle waist stretch.

6. HIPS

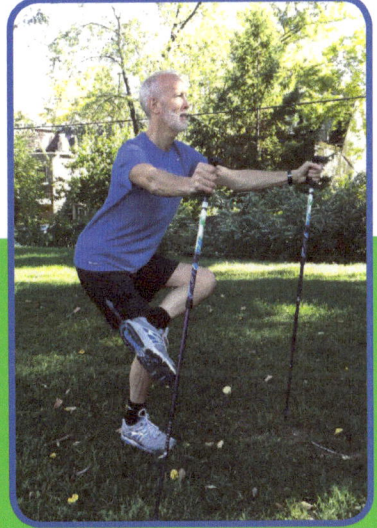

With your poles in front for balance, cross one ankle over the opposite thigh and sit your hips back and down.

1. MY POLES KEEP SLIPPING BACK

This common problem faced by beginners is annoying because when boot tips slip you don't have the traction required to push yourself forward. Fortunately the fix is simple: swing your handles up just an inch higher in front of you. This will put more surface area of your boot tips on the ground. Many people find that just the pole on their non-dominant (weaker and less-coordinated) side slips. It thinks it's swinging all the way up to the handshake position, but it really isn't.

2. I CAN'T KEEP MY ARMS STRAIGHT

Keep practising! Remember that they shouldn't be ramrod straight–just as long as possible with the swing from the shoulders and not the elbows. Try these drills: 1) Practise the arm swing on its own in a stationary position; swing your arms like long pendulums (keeping the boot tips off the ground). Find a large window to check your technique.   2) When you walk down a long hallway or across a parking lot without poles, practise your Nordic walking posture and arm swing with a pair of invisible poles.

3. MY POLES ARE STILL SLIPPING BACK!

Check the treads on your boot tips. If you use your poles regularly, you'll need to replace them every six to 12 months. Like car tires, they slip and slide when they become smooth.

4. MY BOOT TIPS BOUNCE

Press more firmly on the Ledge. This connects the boot tip more firmly to the ground and stops the bounce.

5. I'M DRAGGING MY BOOT TIPS INSTEAD OF LIFTING AND PLANTING THEM

Listen to your boot tips. Try to change the noise they make from a dragging sound to a planting sound. Pretend that you're squishing ants that are on the road with each planting of your boot tips. Remember that it's just a small lift, about one centimetre off the ground.

Easy Fixes

Simple solutions for the most common Nordic walking annoyances

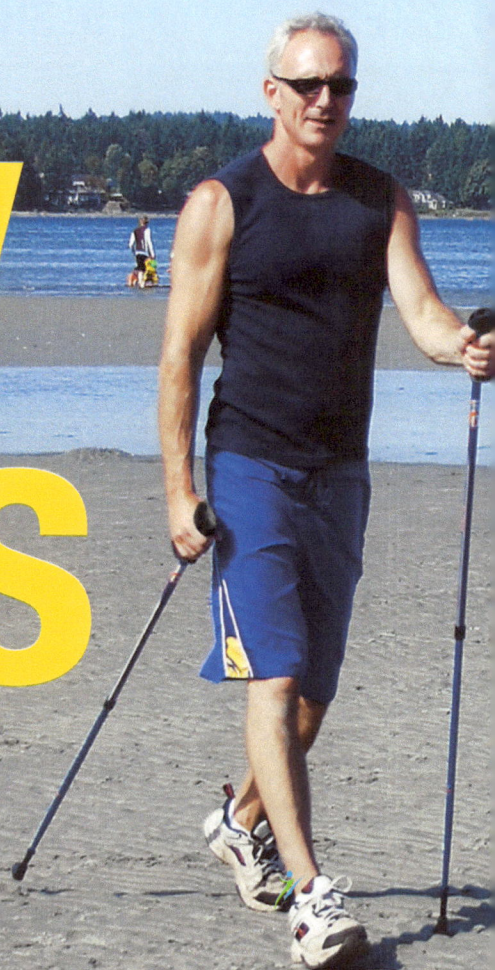

. I DON'T REALLY FEEL MY ABS TIGHTENING

Try this: Stand tall by lengthening from your waist. Now imagine how your core would react if someone was going to vigorously tickle you on both sides of your ribcage. Likely it would tighten and brace in anticipation. This is the sensation you want as you Nordic walk; feel your core muscles tighten each time you press on the Ledge and drive your thumbs to your sides.

7. I DON'T THINK I HAVE THE RIGHT RHYTHM

For every heel plant there is a simultaneous pole plant. Practise this by walking very slowly and somewhat robotically, feeling your opposite heel and boot tip land together each time.

8. I'M A BIT OVER- WHELMED

Try walking with one pole; concentrate on just that one pole, one arm and the opposite leg. Then, practise with just the other pole. Eventually, try walking with both poles. Be patient, keep practising and enjoy the learning process!

9. I CAN'T GET MY HANDS TO RETURN TO THE SIDES OF MY THIGHS

Take a longer step, which will take the sides of your thighs to your hands. If your stride feels awkwardly long, adjust the length while continuing to keep the thighs coming to the hands.

10. THE FRONT OF MY SHOULDERS AND FRONT OF MY ARMS ARE REALLY TIRED

Relax your grip a bit more. Put more emphasis on the pushing down and back (with your hands and arms) phase than the swinging (your hands and arms) up and forward phase.

11. I'M NOT SURE WHAT TO DO WITH MY LEGS

Just keep your legs in sync with your arms. Put your arms and upper body in charge of moving you forward; let the legs come along for the ride.

12. I FIND IT HARD TO GET BACK ON TRACK WHEN I LOSE THE RHYTHM

Relax your arms and drag your poles for a minute or two, letting your arms swing naturally. Then gradually move back into the Nordic walking technique. Or stop for a stretch and a drink, and then start again refreshed.

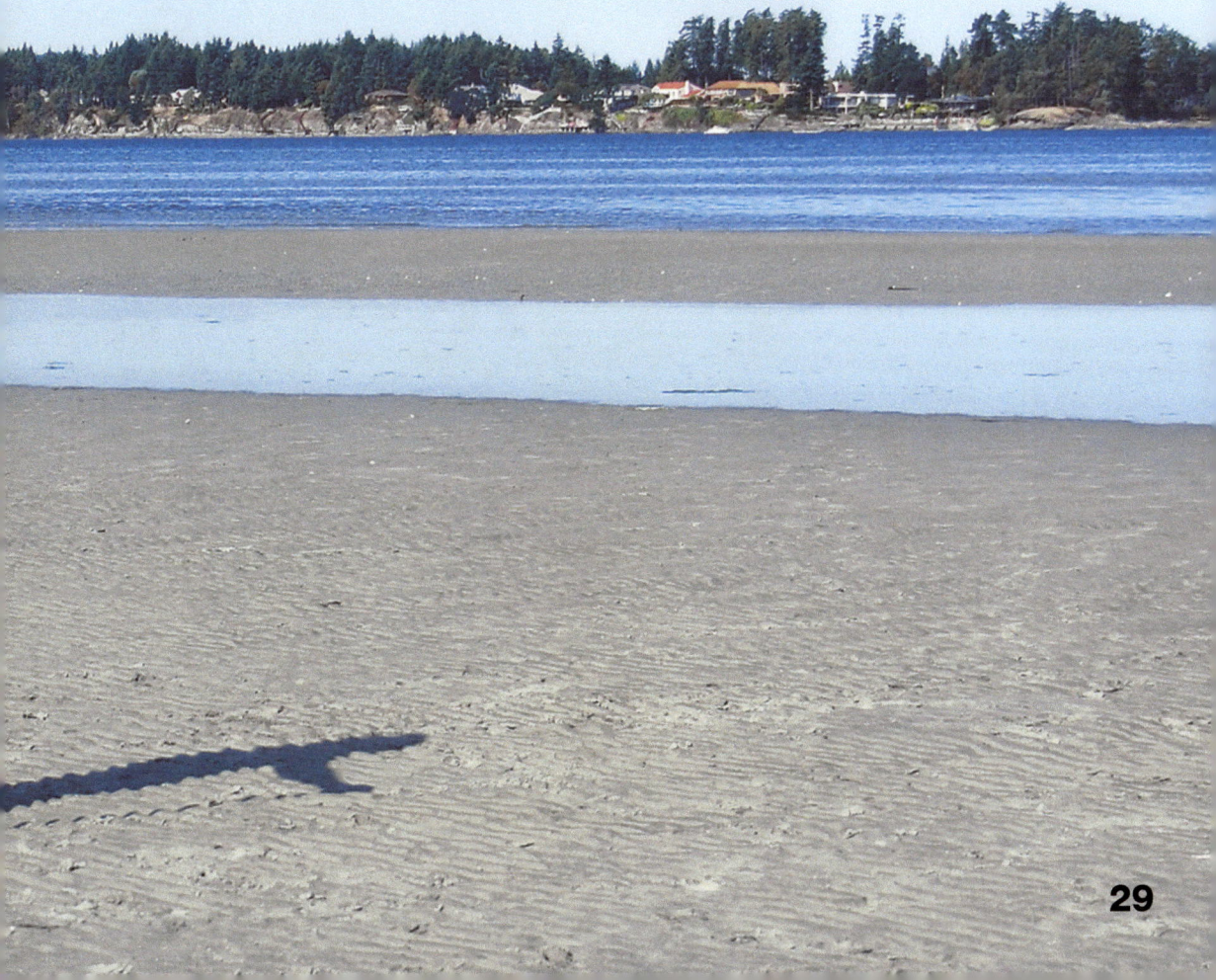

Nordic Walking Secrets That Really Work

1 DON'T LOSE YOUR CLIP

Push the clip (that holds your poles together) to the very top of the pole, and then point it away from your body. This prevents it from hitting your thigh as you walk and possibly detaching.

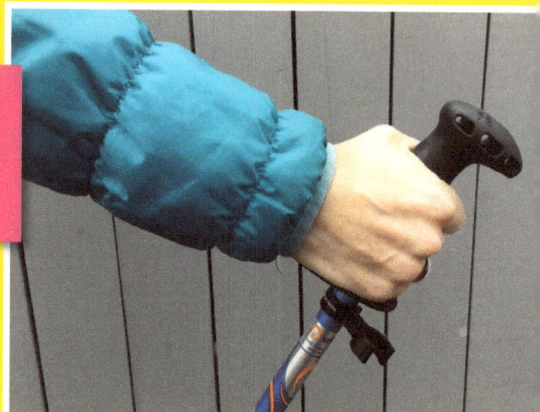

2 SOLVE THE FLAPPING JACKET PROBLEM

When you tie your jacket around your waist, zip it up first before you tie it on. This keeps it tucked neatly behind you and prevents it from getting tangled with your swinging arms and poles.

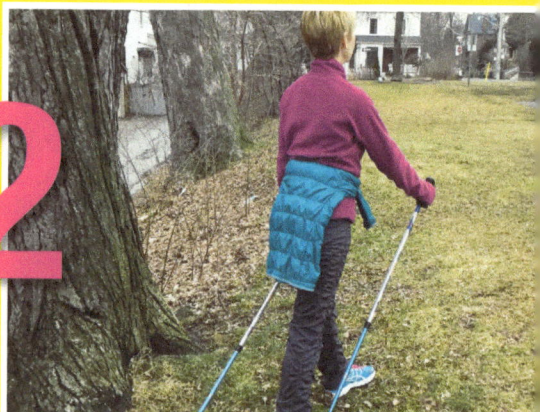

3 KEEP IT CLEAN

Keep your hands and pockets mud-free by inserting your hand into a small plastic bag when handling your boot tips. Dog owners will be familiar with this trick!

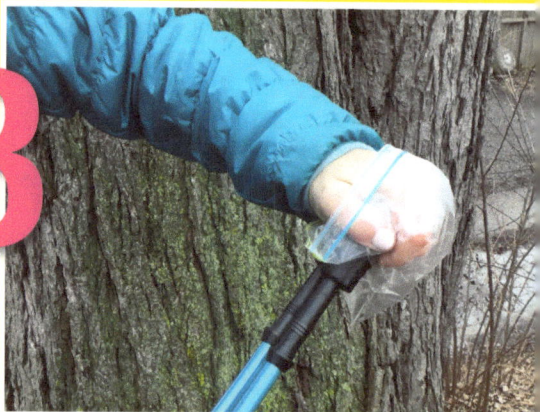

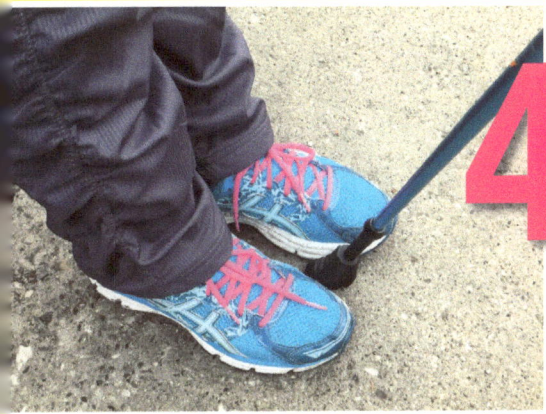

4 ADJUST YOUR BOOT TIPS QUICKLY AND HANDS-FREE

Do as the pros do: when a boot tip is out of alignment, turn the entire pole so the boot tip faces backwards and anchor it between your feet. Then rotate the handle so the R or L is at the top.

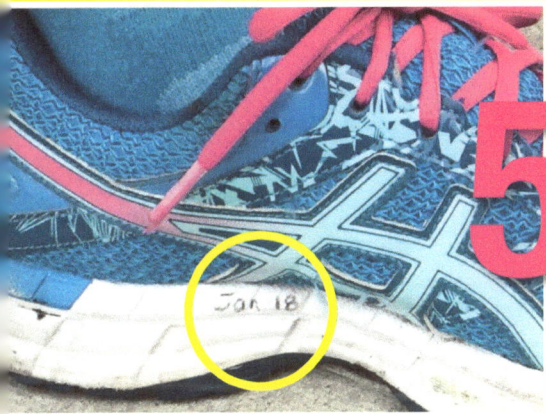

5 GO SHOPPING

Walking and running shoes should be replaced about every 500 kilometres or once a year. To remember the purchase date, write it on the outside instep of one shoe.

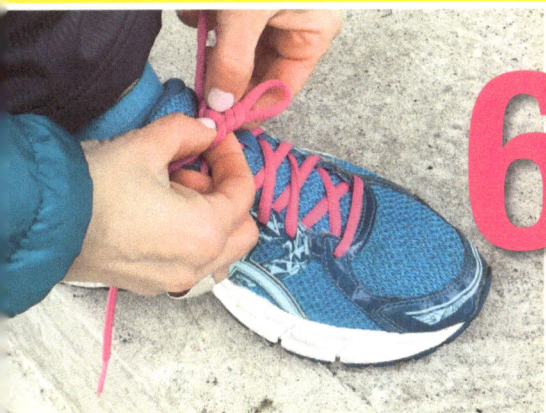

6 SHOELACES GUARAN-TEED TO NEVER UNDO

Tie your laces this way: start as you would normally by tying an overhand knot and then making a bunny ear and wrapping the long lace around it once. Here is what's different: wrap the lace around a second time, and then finish the bow.

GET FIT WITH FIDO

It's fun and practical to include your dog in your workouts. UK-based Janine Lewis teaches "canicross," the sport of cross country exercising while attached to your dog. She offers these suggestions to make Nordic walking with your four-legged friend a pleasant experience for you both.

1 Don't let the poles come close to or touch your dog. If you use proper Nordic walking technique, keeping your poles angled back at 45 degrees, this shouldn't be an issue. You want your dog relaxed around your poles, not afraid of them.

2 Find a leash system that works for you. With one popular system, the owner wears a waist belt, the dog wears a harness and you are attached to each other via a two-metre bungee line.

3 Leave treats at home. Carrying delicious-smelling treats in your pockets will likely distract your dog. Instead, reward good behaviour at the end of the walk and with something that you offer only after Nordic walking.

4 Use one-word commands. Guide your dog with a command of, for example, "left" or "right" rather than using full sentences.

5 React to your dog's body language. To prevent your dog from zigzagging and possibly pulling you off balance, try a command of "leave it" when the nose goes down to scent or to the side. When the nose is back up and on track give reinforcement with a happy voice.

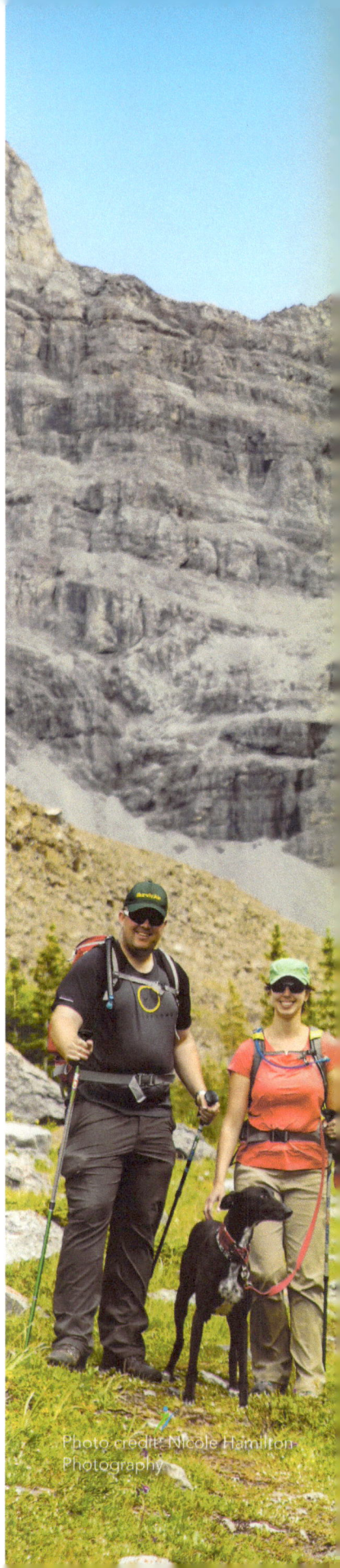

Photo credit: Nicole Hamilton Photography

WHICH STRATEGIES & DOG LEASH WORK BEST FOR YOU?

"I use a hands-free runner's leash around my hips to Nordic walk with my six-year-old Golden Retriever Codie. The leash has an elasticized portion, so there is some give if he decides to sniff along the way. I prefer him to stay slightly behind me in a heel position and my arm in front of the leash. For our first few walks, I just carried the poles because he was afraid of them. I also recommend starting in familiar surroundings with minimal distractions."
Marianne Leung
Markham, Ont.

"Good heeling training is a huge step in the right direction to successful Nordic walking with your dog. With my black Labrador Retriever Whisper, I use my training leash looped through the belt of my waist pack and position it in my mid-back. Now that Whisper is more advanced in her obedience training, our walks are worry-free."
Fran Betts
Wallaceburg, Ont.

"The heel position definitely doesn't work for our very energetic three-year-old Lab mix Dixie who loves to pull! She is very leery of moving objects that come close to her. For trail walks with poles I have her on an Easy Walk harness—which rests across her chest instead of around her throat—which I wear around my waist. She walks out in front of me. She occasionally veers to the side, but a pole coming in from the outside to push the leash back to the middle easily gets her back on course."
Kari Galasso
Kingston, Ont.

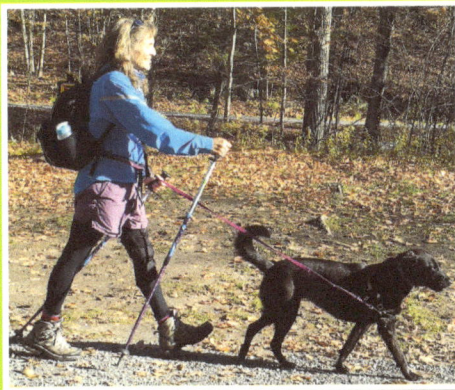

FAQS

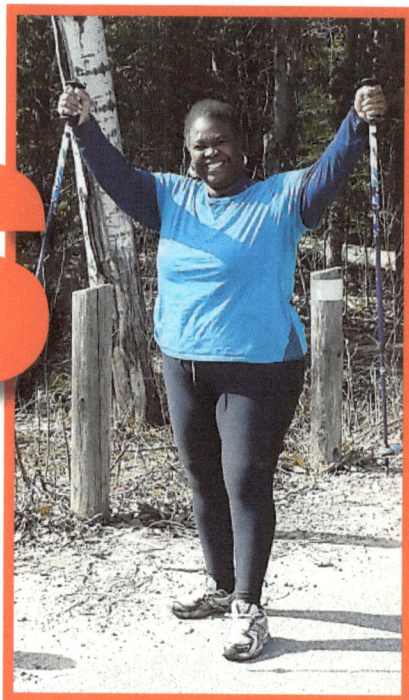

Answers to the most frequently asked questions about Nordic walking

1. **When do I take off the boot tips and use the carbide tips?**
The boot tips are used on hard surfaces, such as sidewalks and asphalt, while the carbide tips (under the boot tips) are for soft surfaces, such as dirt trails, soft snow and gravel. There is no wrong choice; choose the option that provides the best traction and shock absorption for the surface.

2. **How long will it take me to become a proficient Nordic walker?**
Like any new skill, practise makes perfect. Some people feel confident and comfortable after just a few outings or classes, while others take much longer to perfect their technique. Enjoy the journey!

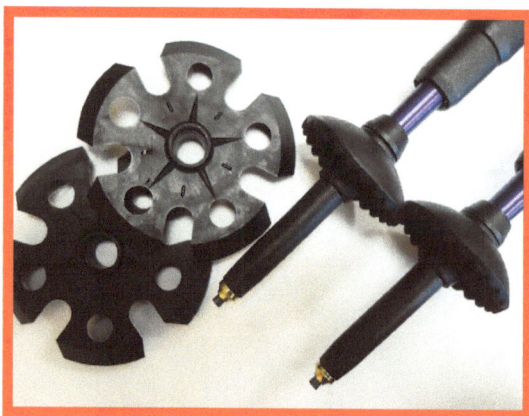

3. **Why do some poles have straps and some don't?**
Research shows that Nordic walking is a safe activity, but the most frequent injury is 'skier's thumb,' a thumb dislocation or sprain that occurs when a person falls with an open hand onto the handle of a pole. The founders of Urban Poling wanted to avoid this risk, and they also preferred the ease-of-use of the strapless system.

4. **Now that I'm exercising more regularly, how can I prevent leg cramps that I occasionally get in bed?**
Before you go to bed, stretch the muscles that tend to cramp (see page 28). Hold each stretch for 30–60 seconds, and perform it at least twice on each leg.

5. **If I'm not very fit, sporty or coordinated, can I be successful at Nordic walking?**
Yes! Nordic walkers come in all shapes, ages, sizes and fitness levels.

6. **How does the technique of a beginner and an advanced Nordic walker differ?**
Nordic walking is similar to many other physical activities—such as swimming, tennis, running and dancing—in that the basic technique is the same for everyone. Advanced participants simply move faster and with more precise technique and confidence.

7. What does a Nordic walking class look like? Why should I take one?

Classes from a certified Nordic walking instructor are the quickest way to learn. Check the "Find a Class" link on the "Education" tab at www.urban-poling.com. Class design varies, but most classes are 45–60 minutes and include a warm-up and cool down stretching, ongoing technique instruction and perhaps some stationary exercises using the poles. Instructors are great motivators who often help you to walk a little further, a little faster or with better style than you would if you were on your own.

8. Can I use my poles in snow, on the beach, for downhill skiing, for mall walking or on an indoor track?

Yes to all of these locations, (but please don't use them on a treadmill)! Add snow baskets for snow-shoeing, downhill skiing and walking in deep snow. For indoor Nordic walking, check the floor surface to be sure it's not too slippery for your boot tips.

9. I have poor balance and lack confidence while walking. Are Nordic walking poles the best choice for me?

Urban Poling's Activator poles and the Activator walking technique, both designed to provide balance and stability, may be a better option (visit www.urbanpoling.com).

10. Can I use my hiking/trekking/tramping poles in place of Nordic walking poles?

Sorry, no. Though they might look similar at first glance, each type of pole is designed specifically to fit its intended use.

Hiking/trekking poles are designed to *minimize* energy expenditure by creating stability and taking stress off the hips and knees. The poles are usually held vertically in front of the body; the handles often have finger-grooves and a loop strap to help prevent dropping the poles; and they don't have rubber tips since they're not used on pavement. (Any round plastic tips are to protect the tips when they're being stored or transported.) There is no specific walking technique to learn.

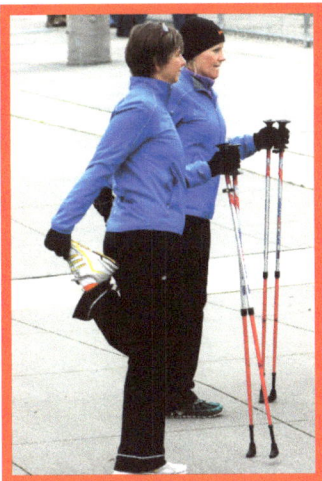

Nordic walking poles are designed to *maximize* energy expenditure by actively engaging your upper body with a full arm swing and a "plant, push, propel" action. The poles are held at a 45 degree angle with the tips always angled behind your body. Urban Poling brand handles are strapless and have a large Ledge on the base of a thick handle where walkers exert pressure. A second style of Nordic walking poles has straps (that are often like mini-gloves) where pressure is exerted. Both strapless and strap-style Nordic walking poles have detachable rubber boot-shaped tips for walking on hard surfaces, such as pavement.

11. Why do I see some Nordic walkers walking with technique that is different than described here?

Unfortunately, some people don't seek out training or do any research at all regarding proper technique. As a result, it's unlikely they'll achieve the fitness and health benefits that people with good Nordic walking technique achieve.

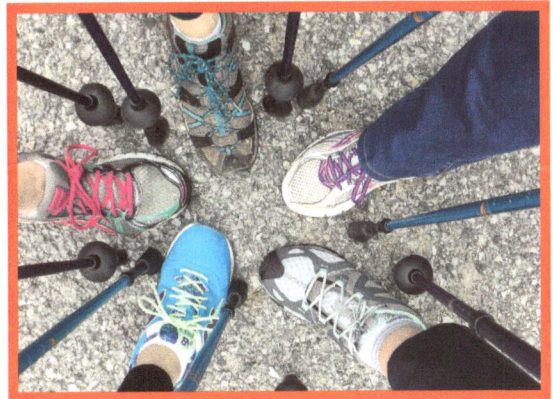

12. Do I really need an athletic shoe expert to size me up?

Yes! Good quality shoes, which will provide proper arch support and address the unique needs of your feet, add immensely to the enjoyment of any physical activity.

(Continues on next page)

13. **Do I really need high-tech fitness clothes?**
Any comfortable clothes will be just fine. But if you walk substantial distances or perspire when you Nordic walk, the smooth seams, non-constricting designs and fabrics that wick away sweat are well worth the investment.

14. **How important is a warm-up and cool down?** Unless you have issues with your joints, a warm-up is usually not necessary. However, cooldown stretching is very important to keep your muscles long and your joints mobile.

15. **Can I achieve the body of my dreams with Nordic walking?**
Nordic walking will boost your health and fitness in numerous ways, but a healthy diet is very important if weight loss is a key goal.

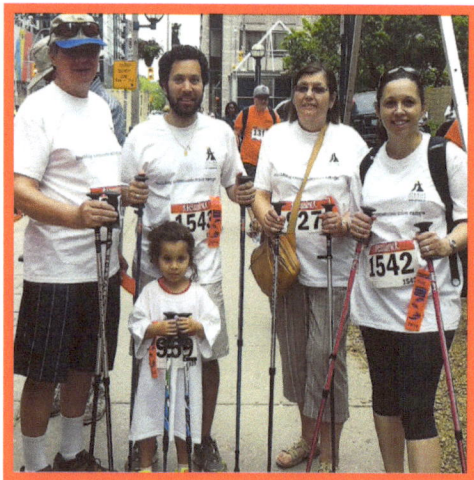

16. **Can I take my poles in race event?**
Many events happily accept Nordic walkers. Check each race event's fine print, or join in with the walkers being careful to stay to the back of the crowd and to the side so your poles aren't a hazard.

17. **How long should a Nordic walk be?**
Nordic walking requires more energy than standard walking. The first few times out, try about one-third of the time you typically walk without poles. Evaluate how you feel afterwards, and then adjust the time accordingly for future Nordic walks.

18. **What's the biggest technique mistake that people make?**
Many people find it challenging to keep their arms long and extended as they walk. Or as they tire or lose focus, the swinging starts to come from the elbows instead of the shoulders and the upper arms stop moving.

19. **When should I replace my boot tips?**
Check the tread on your boot tips regularly. Like car tires, they lose their traction over time. Good boot tips have lots of tread, are a bit springy and are less likely to slip when you plant them. People with good technique—who plant their boot tips rather than dragging them—find their boot tips last much longer. You will likely need to replace them every 6–12 months, depending on how frequently you Nordic walk and the quality of your technique.

20. **What can I do if I feel a bit self-conscious exercising with my poles?**
Go with a friend or a group of friends. There are more people every day taking up the activity. Remember that fifteen years ago inline skaters garnered lots of attention, but today no one takes notice as they whiz by.

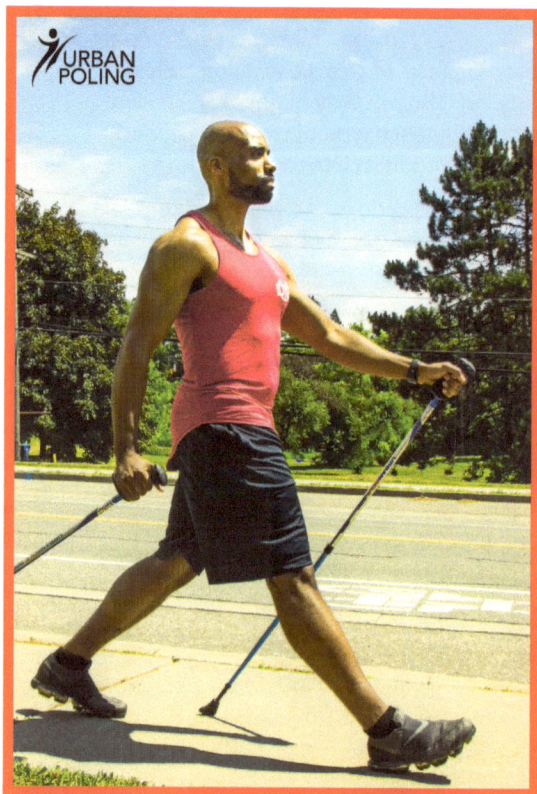

ONE OF THE **BEST MOMENTS** IN LIFE IS REALIZING THAT TWO WEEKS AGO YOUR BODY COULDN'T DO WHAT IT JUST DID.

NORDIC WALKING as MEDICINE

If you're recovering from surgery or are living with a chronic health condition*, Nordic walking can be a powerful tonic. Consider this advice from top fitness and healthcare professionals.

1 If you've been inactive and are just starting with poles, start very slowly. My clients with arthritis often overdo it by Nordic walking for too long or too fast the first time because they're so happy to be moving again and without pain.

Jessica Lewgood
kinesiologist
Estevan, Saskatchewan

2 Learn to recognize the difference between discomfort and pain. If Nordic walking hurts, don't do it. But if it is discomfort, try working through it. If you're in pain a few hours later, address the situation then.

Don Ferguson
older adults fitness instructor
Ottawa

* For example: arthritis, diabetes, heart disease, stroke, fibromyalgia, chronic pain, soft tissue injury, depression and anxiety.

3 Try not to look down in front of your feet as you walk. Your balance system functions optimally when your head is up and your eyes are looking ahead. This head position also helps to facilitate an upright posture.

Sue Colbourne
occupational therapist
Duncan, B.C.

4 Consider an indoor track. The flat smooth surface feels great on the joints and lets you walk without leaving the comfort and security of the building. Walk both clockwise and counter clockwise—it varies the scenery and is best for your knees.

Don Ferguson
older adults fitness instructor
Ottawa

5 If you're scheduled for surgery, both the ACTIVATOR® poles and Nordic walking poles are ideal for "prehab." Using the poles to improve your fitness level before you undergo surgery can greatly speed your recovery.

Mandy Shintani
occupational therapist
Vancouver

6 In the beginning, your arms may get very tired. If so, instead of pressing on the Ledge with every arm swing, try concentrating on the right arm for 10 presses, the left arm for 10 presses, and then use both arms for 10 presses.

Cathy McNorgan
physiotherapist
Wellesley, Ont.

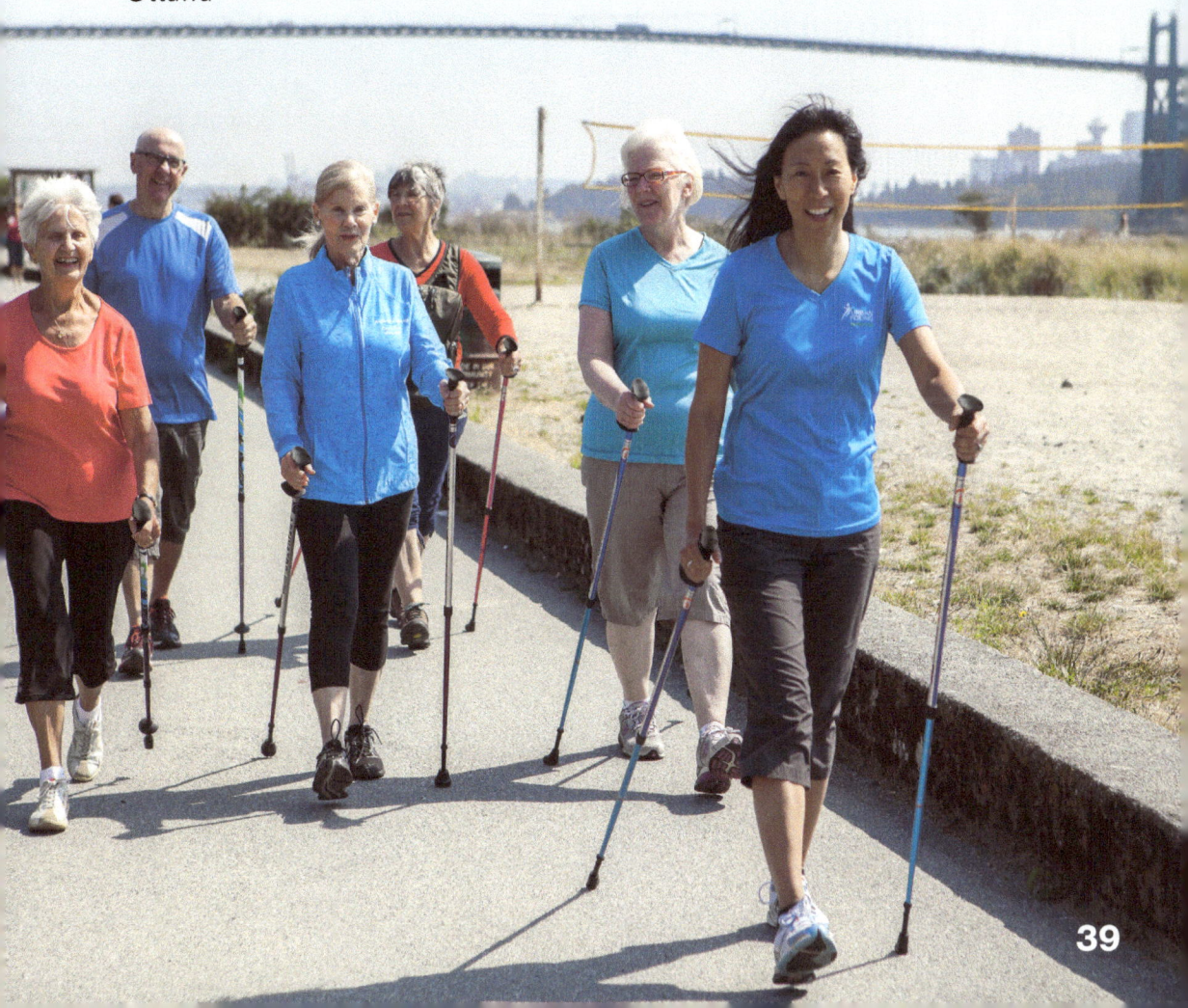

SPRING BACK INTO ACTION WITH PRE-HAB

The secret to speedy post-surgery recovery is all about poles

Before her hip replacement surgery Wendy Crean couldn't manage a stroll around the block, and grocery shopping was out of the question.

"Walking felt like torture," says the retired nurse from Toronto.

But just three months post-surgery, her health and mobility had skyrocketed. She was pain-free and back to leading an active life.

Crean credits much of her speedy recovery to "pre-hab"–a proactive pre-surgery approach to improving the body's overall function and resilience–using her Nordic walking poles.

"Before my surgery, regular walking was too painful, but with my poles I could really move along," says Crean, whose pre-hab involved regular 30-minute walks with her poles in a local park with one or two rest stops along the way. "The poles relieved the pain, they gave me confidence and I felt really safe. I was moving my arms, I was out in the fresh air, and I felt like million bucks."

Pre-hab has long been recommended by physiotherapists for patients undergoing planned surgeries, such as hip and knee replacements, says Dolores Langford, physiotherapy practice coordinator at Vancouver Coastal Health.

Langford is a big fan of Nordic walking for her clients. "Without the poles, pain prevents people from being active," she says. "But the poles take pressure off your joints which reduces pain and increases walking tolerance and confidence. People can walk further with them plus use them to help with their balance and strengthening exercises."

> **"Joint replacement surgery is like running a marathon."**
>
> **Dolores Langford**
> *physiotherapist & Urban Poling certified instructor*

She also appreciates Urban Poling's large easy-to-hold handles that don't aggravate arthritic fingers.

"I tell my clients that joint replacement surgery is like running a marathon," says Langford. "If you prepare early and properly, you'll come out stronger on the other side and bounce back much quicker."

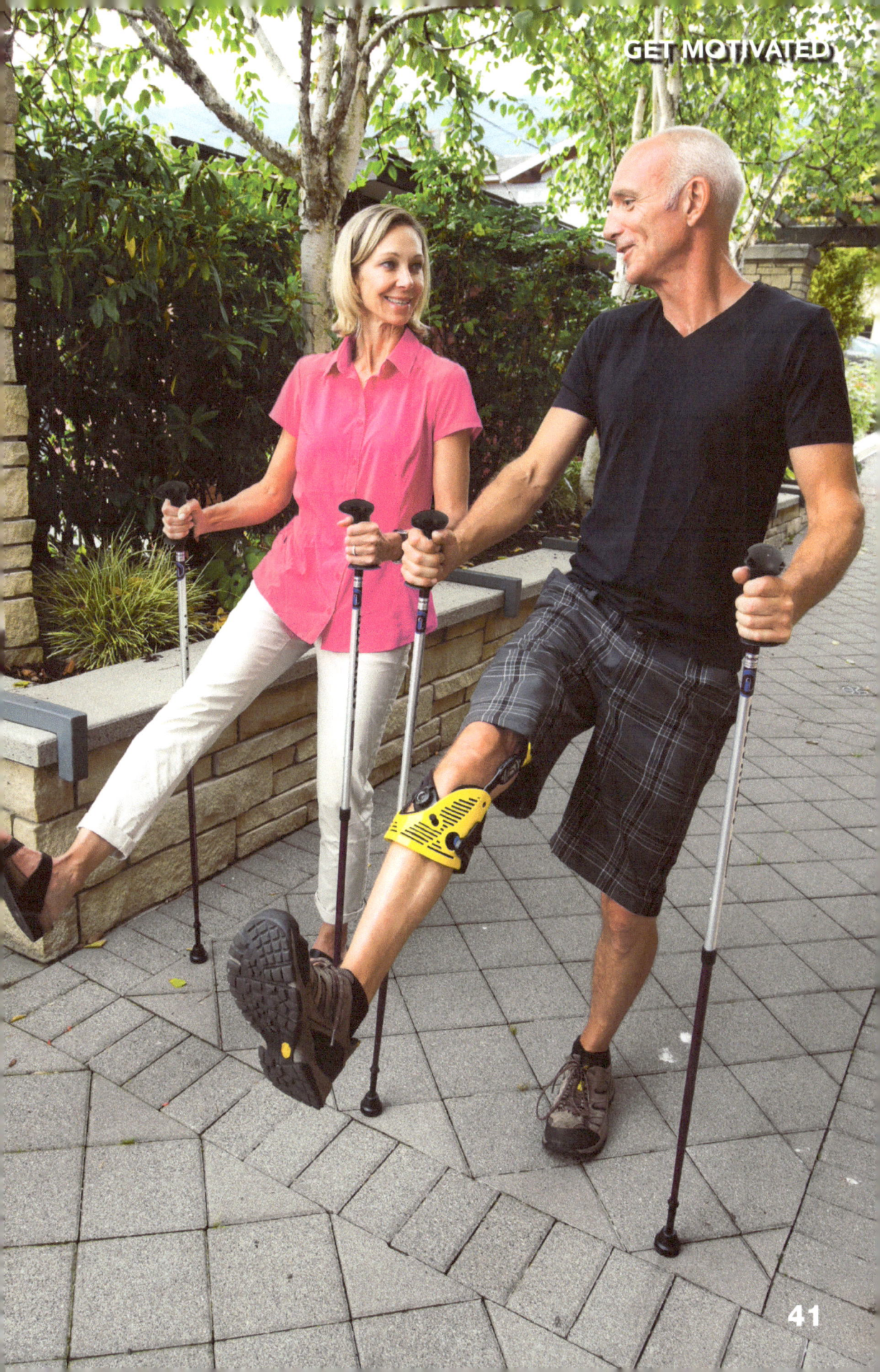

WALKING

I Nordic Walked for 30 Consecutive Days and Here's What Happened

TALL

Nordic walker: Blayne Mackey
City: Kingston, Ontario
Age: 68
Occupation: retired
Nordic walking experience: 2 years

Honestly, did you walk 30 days in a row?

Yes! It was tempting to stay indoors on some of the rainy and blustery days, but I really wanted the satisfaction of meeting the challenge. So I grabbed my poles and went out anyway, even if it was just for a short walk.

How long were your walks?

I tried to Nordic walk 2.5 kilometres on three days, 5 kilometres on other three days and 7.5 kilometres for the last day. A few rainy-day walks were shorter, but I still got out there. On one really hectic day, instead of cancelling, I cut the walk to 20 minutes. It was a beautiful walk and really reduced the pressures of that busy day.

How's retired life?

Since I retired five years ago, I've had time to put a greater focus on my health. I've lost 40 pounds by exercising regularly and switching to a vegan diet. I'm currently attending Weight Watchers with a goal to lose 15 more pounds. I've been stuck at 190 for a while now, but I feel great. I lost two pounds during this challenge, so hopefully the trend will continue.

Was it difficult to keep on track during your beach vacation?

Not at all. At low tide there was a good stretch of beautiful beach with hard packed sand, crashing waves and folks out looking for shells. I used my poles without the boot tips. At high tide I walked on neighbourhood sidewalks. A couple of gardeners asked if I was looking for snow. I definitely was not—it was nice to be in warm weather and wearing shorts and a T-shirt in November!

What I Learned

1. When I walk longer than 60 minutes, I need a snack and drink. A mix of raisins and peanuts and some chocolate milk work well to keep up my energy.

2. Hiking boots are best for trail walking because they keep out small stones that get kicked up. For asphalt and concrete sidewalks, running shoes are best because they're lighter and give better traction.

3. It's nice to join an instructor-led group once a week. Our local Urban Poling instructor, Kari Galasso, noticed that my posture was off and suggested lengthening my poles to my full height (versus two inches lower as recommended for beginners). Now I'm standing more upright. The class also includes a warm up and cooldown stretching, which I often omit when I'm on my own.

4. Walking in the rain is actually pleasant when you wear rain gear.

5. Compared to regular walking, which I find isn't challenging enough, I experience a 20 percent increase in heart rate when using my poles. I'm a data wonk, so I track my heart rate and other workout details using a Polar M400 watch and chest strap.

6. A great Nordic walk can easily be undone by a poor meal. I'm reading *The Mindful Diet: How to Transform Your Relationship with Food for Lasting Weight Loss and Vibrant Health* by Ruth Wolever and finding it very informative.

Work It In

Struggle finding time to exercise?
A new-ish Nordic walker shares her insights

Be realistic

I tried committing to Nordic walking every day, but it sometimes felt more like a chore than a pleasure. Instead, I take long walks four to five times a week. This way I feel good about my accomplishments at the end of the week.

Don't let a hectic schedule be a roadblock

Saturdays are full of errands with my husband, and we often have guests for dinner and sometimes for the weekend. But by walking early in the morning, I still manage to get in a 20-40 minute workout. If it's a short walk, I increase my speed.

Always think form

I've been trying to increase my speed to burn more calories. When I walk very quickly for one hour with good technique, I feel strong, refreshed and pleased with myself at the end of a session. On days when I move at a more leisurely pace, I compensate by walking for a longer time.

Have fun with a tracker

It excites me when my pedometer shows 10,000 steps by mid-afternoon. I also love comparing data. For example, after a summer of little exercise (due to intense heat), my pedometer showed that in the beginning it took me two hours to walk a favourite 7.1 km. route, and just one week later it took 10 minutes less.

Move all year round

I got started by signing up for a nine-week series of classes in the middle of last winter. I loved it! There was a great group of folks who participated, and it made the season more enjoyable. We even poled on the very cold days.

Get creative

Sometimes I drive into town with my husband and then walk home (7.8 km.), which takes about 1.75 hours. For these long walks, my goal is to just cover the distance and to not focus too much on time. When I'm having my car serviced, instead of sitting and waiting, I take my poles with me and go for a walk.

Be mindful of the benefits

Thanks to a focus on regular Nordic walking and eating well, I lost four pounds last month, I'm sleeping better, and my walking pace and stamina have increased.

Keep it all in perspective

This year I Nordic walked after attending a cold and windy Remembrance Day ceremony. I didn't want to, but I rationalized that given the sacrifices of our Armed Forces it was the least I could do. It was miserable and tiring, but I was proud of myself for walking 40 minutes.

"

I'm tired after my Nordic walks, but it's that satisfying tired that comes from knowing I've done something good for myself.

"

THE GAME CHANGER

As Nordic walking helps him lose weight, de-stress and battle cancer, Richard Lavery pays it forward by teaching others

Photo credit: Doug Bingham

I have been reasonably active for most of my adult life–running, taking exercise classes, skiing and walking. But over the years my activity level declined while my couch time increased. I noticed my muscle mass, strength and energy waning, my waistline expanding and my core sagging. In a quest to rediscover my fitness, I found that ordinary walking just wasn't enough. I didn't want to go to a gym, so my body bagged and sagged and lost its agility and power.

But then I discovered Nordic walking, and ever since it has been my key activity and saviour. It provides a challenging workout, eases life's daily stresses and gives me the opportunity to enjoy the beauty of my hometown.

It all started in 2015, when I took a seniors exercise instructor course and then a Nordic walking instructor certification course offered by Urban Poling. Within hours of my introduction to Nordic walking, it was a love affair.
Never had I done an activity that presented such a wide

> **Like most guys, I have two very reticent left feet and coordination on the minus scale. But, fortunately, I also have an enthusiastic attitude.**

range of physical demands. I believe it is the almost perfect physical activity. If you Nordic walk daily, within just weeks you will feel profound effects: strength, agility and flexibility will return to your neck, shoulders, arms, wrists, upper and lower back, chest and abs. Your posture will be noticeably more upright, your shoulders back and abs tightened.

After my first few Nordic walks, I needed to follow up with anti-inflammatories to ease the ache from a long-ago skiing injury. But then the veil of pain receded and the functionality of my shoulder returned, along with more mobility in my neck. My increased level of fitness has been a huge bonus. I feel like my overall muscle mass has increased at least 10 percent—no small feat. In six months I have snugged down my belt three inches and lost ten pounds.

Unfortunately, two years ago I was diagnosed with prostate cancer. For those who have experienced serious illness, injury or major difficulty in your life, you know how your stress level dramatically increases.

Once again, Nordic walking has been my game changer. It is a walking meditation that I use to aggressively challenge my physical being as my spiritual self seeks some relative peace. It enables me to sort through raging emotions and to tame the anxiety beast. It keeps my body and my inner self strong to fight this invasive disease.

My enthusiasm also extends to teaching others. I have taught people from their fifties to their eighties and those struggling with balance, weight, arthritis, diabetes, and post-surgery and rehabilitation issues.

Time takes its toll, but a simple pair of poles can help you fight back.

Get Moving to Fight Depression

For Dolly Hayes, Nordic walking proves to be just what the doctor ordered

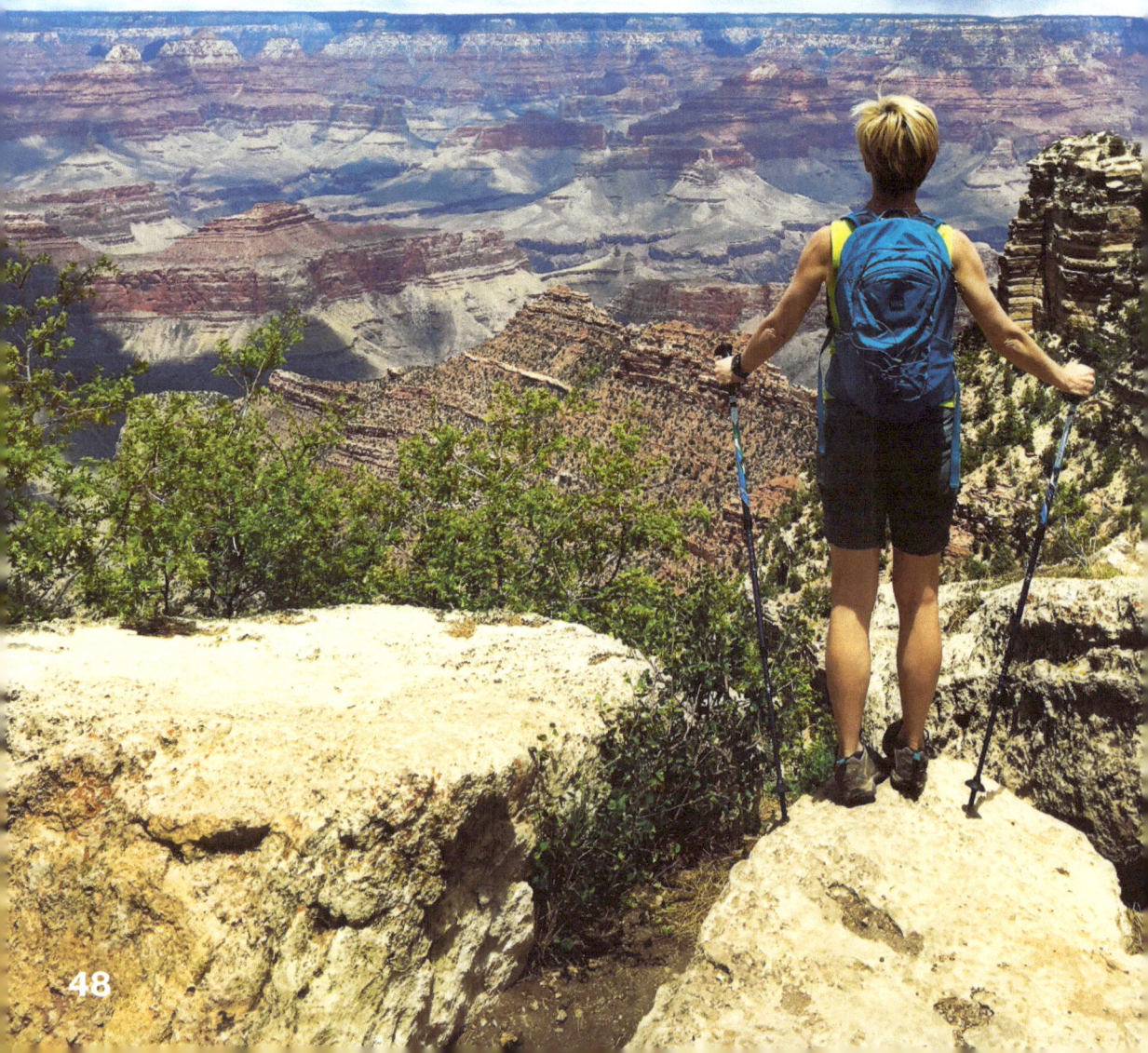

In 1998 I was diagnosed with clinical depression, and then in 2004 I lost my husband after a long struggle with cancer. Add to this an assortment of other stressors, and before I knew it I was 100 pounds overweight.

I realized things had to change when one day I found it impossible to complete even simple chores around the house. My knees were killing me and my blood pressure was up. I knew it was time to make some drastic changes.

I had tried walking with a friend, but it was too painful. An orthopaedic surgeon suggested surgery. I opted for a cortisone shot instead, but it only decreased the pain temporarily.

Nordic walking to the rescue

Then one day, two friends—one being a physiotherapist and Urban Poling-certified instructor—introduced me to Nordic walking. At first it was very awkward, and I couldn't quite get the rhythm. But they encouraged me to keep at it, and suddenly it felt wonderful. In fact, I loved it almost immediately because the poles took a tremendous amount of pressure off my knees.

I started poling regularly,

> ## "
> ## To celebrate my newfound health and lifestyle, I went on a fantastic holiday to Arizona and the Grand Canyon where my friends and I enjoyed long Nordic walks through spectacular scenery.
> ## "

gradually increasing my workouts from three 20- to 30-minute sessions per week to three 60-minute sessions.

At about the same time, I started following the Weight Watchers program. Recording my daily food intake, attending the weekly meetings and receiving lots of encouragement from the leader, group participants and my children helped me stick with it.

As time progressed, instead of socializing over food I started scheduling Nordic walking sessions with my friends. We're still walking together today, and we all love it!

Hard work pays off

I'm very proud of my achievements: I have lost 100 pounds, my knees are now pain-free and I can Nordic walk for two hours straight.

But best of all I now enjoy regular post-workout endorphin highs that help manage my depression and carry me through my day.

Nordic walking combined with healthy eating has been the best possible thing for my mental health. These days my emotions are in check, and I'm able to put a bad day in the past. I know that yesterday was yesterday and that I have the power and the tools to create a better today.

FROM REHAB-ER TO REHAB-EE

When illness stopped her in her tracks, occupational therapist Sue Colbourne was grateful for her Nordic walking poles

As an occupational therapist, I have been recommending Nordic walking to my clients since 2012. In fact, I was so impressed with the poles that I became an Urban Poling master trainer so I could teach my rehab colleagues about Nordic walking's many benefits.

But I gained a new perspective on poling when my husband Guy and I used the poles for our own rehabilitation.

Double trouble

This past spring, I contracted whooping cough, which damages the respiratory system. The cough persists for at least 100 days, with the worst coughing occurring in the first month. This excessive coughing led to a lack of sleep and significant weight loss, culminating in extreme fatigue.

Guy, who has done decades of manual labour, has had several injuries that led to pressure on his spinal cord.

The same day that he was undergoing spinal surgery to prevent permanent paralysis, I was in the hospital's emergency department. I truly thought I was going to die because I was so weak. Walking to the bathroom was all I could manage at that point.

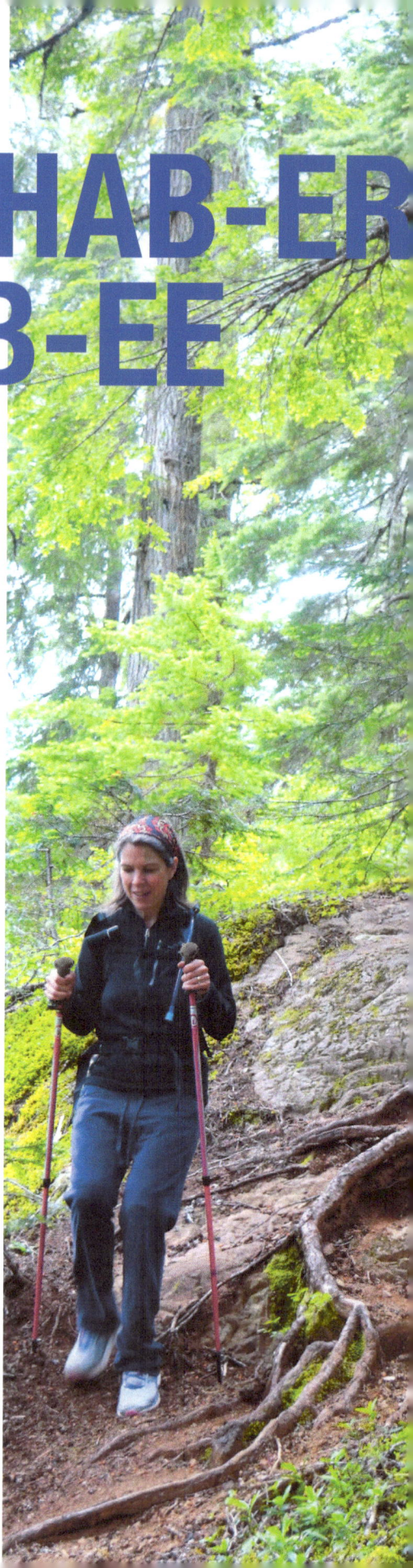

Thankfully, Guy's surgery was successful. But once home, it was clear that he needed to increase his strength and weight-bearing activity to promote the formation of new bone. He also wanted to lose some weight that had accumulated during the previous inactive months.

Getting active again

In the early stages of our rehab, Guy could walk much further with his poles than me. In the beginning, all I could tolerate was a five-minute trip to the mailbox.

Although I have worked with clients for whom fatigue has been a significant issue, I had never personally experienced how debilitating it truly can be. Even taking a shower required hours to recover. I remember thinking how unrealistic some of my expectations had been for my clients.

During the early stage of my illness I couldn't drive, and my cognitive abilities and reaction time were slowed. This made my poles invaluable. I appreciated eventually being able to exercise every morning on the quiet trails near our home.

Hard work, patience and Nordic walking pay off

In time, both of us were able to walk for two hours on flat terrain. Later we progressed to more-challenging hikes where the poles were essential on steeper ground.

As I write this, my rehab is complete. Guy has lost 26 pounds and is starting to woodwork again. And, of course, we continue to use our poles to make further gains in our fitness.

> **" My strength, energy and independence have been renewed. "**

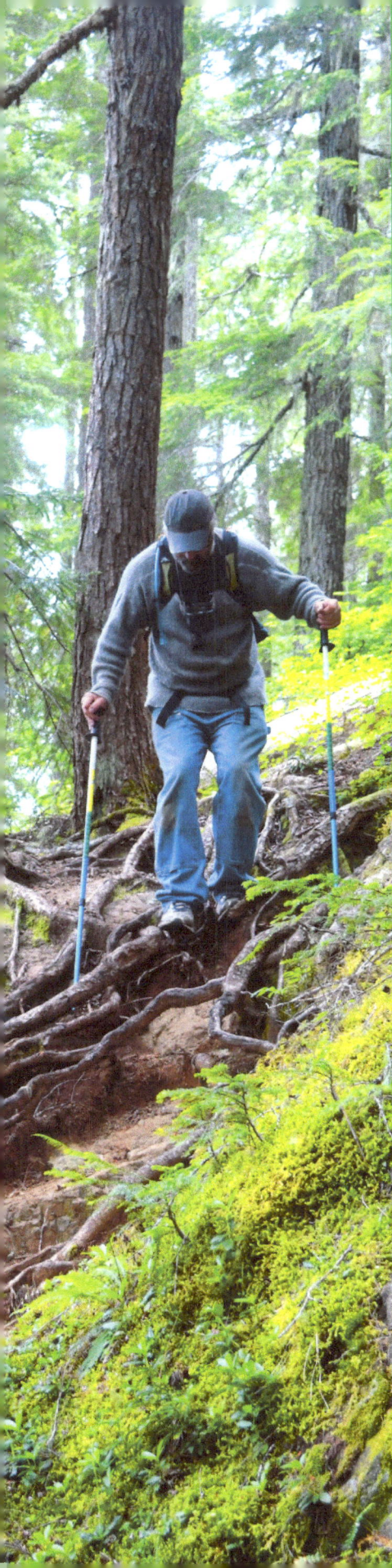

Fight Arthritis with Nordic Walking

Let poles help you outsmart the aches and pains of arthritis

If you have osteoporosis, arthritis or just the simple aches and pains that come with age, your first instinct may be to dial down the physical activity in your life. After all, there's less chance of worsening the pain if you're quietly seated. Isn't there?

This kind of thinking is seriously outdated, says Fran Betts, who is district coordinator of the VON Canada Seniors Exercise and Fall Prevention Program and lives in Wallaceburg, Ontario.

"It can be tempting to stop moving," says Fran, "but exercise helps increase your bone mass, muscle strength and coordination, and it keeps you flexible and limber."

Fran speaks from personal experience. About 17 years ago, the long time fitness instructor was recovering from hip replacement surgery and dealing with the beginnings of arthritis in both feet.

She wanted to get back to teaching fitness classes, but even simple walking was too painful.

"Then I gave a Nordic walking class a try, and to my amazement found that I could walk for longer periods of time with significantly less discomfort," says Fran. "It was fun and easy to learn, and I purchased the fitness poles on the spot."

Starting with short walks, she gradually increased her distance every weekend.

Wise Words About Arthritis

- **In the long term, physical activity will decrease the pain caused by your arthritis. And it can do wonders for your state of mind.**

- **Being active will actually increase your energy levels and let you get more out of your day.**

- **If your activities leave you feeling overly tired, you're probably doing too much too fast.**

"As I became better at the technique, I noticed a change in my posture and in the strength of my core muscles, arms and legs," she says. "A portion of my body weight was being transferred through the poles rather than totally through my feet, which helped ease the foot pain. And the plant-push-propel technique was turning my walks into total body workouts, just as the instructor had promised."

Before she knew it, Fran had poled her way through a 10K fundraiser and become a certified Urban Poling Nordic walking instructor.

"The best news is that with my poles I've been able to get back to walking the Bruce Trail with my husband and our dog," she says. "This was something I thought I might never do again!"

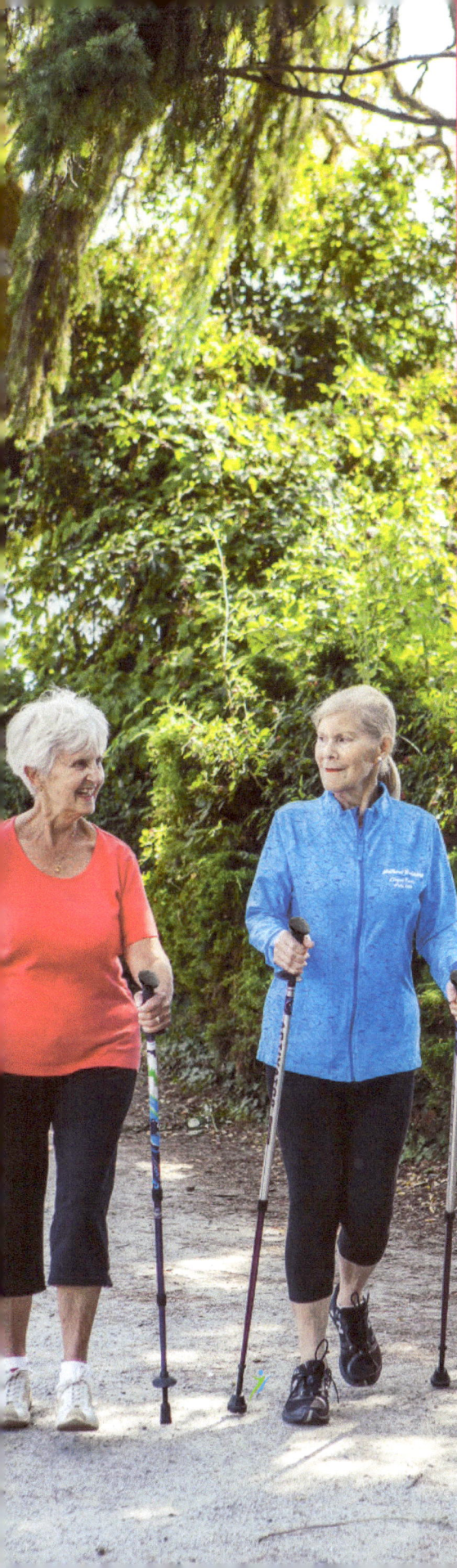

12 REASONS
TO NORDIC WALK
TODAY

1. | I will have the desire to eat healthier foods.

2. | I will be less stressed and anxious.

3. | I will be more mentally alert.

PRIVATE PROPERTY
NO DUMPING
VIOLATORS WILL BE PROSECUTED

4. I will be energized for the rest of the day.

5. I will have a sharper memory.

6. I will lower my risk for a multitude of diseases.

7. I will be doing something just for me.

8. I will feel happier.

9. I will have more confidence.

10. I will be one step closer to my goal.

11. I will sleep better.

12. I will strengthen my muscles and bones.

Mural by Herakut

Pick Up The Pace!

Want to get fitter faster? Ramp up the intensity of your Nordic walking workouts with one (or more) of these strategies.

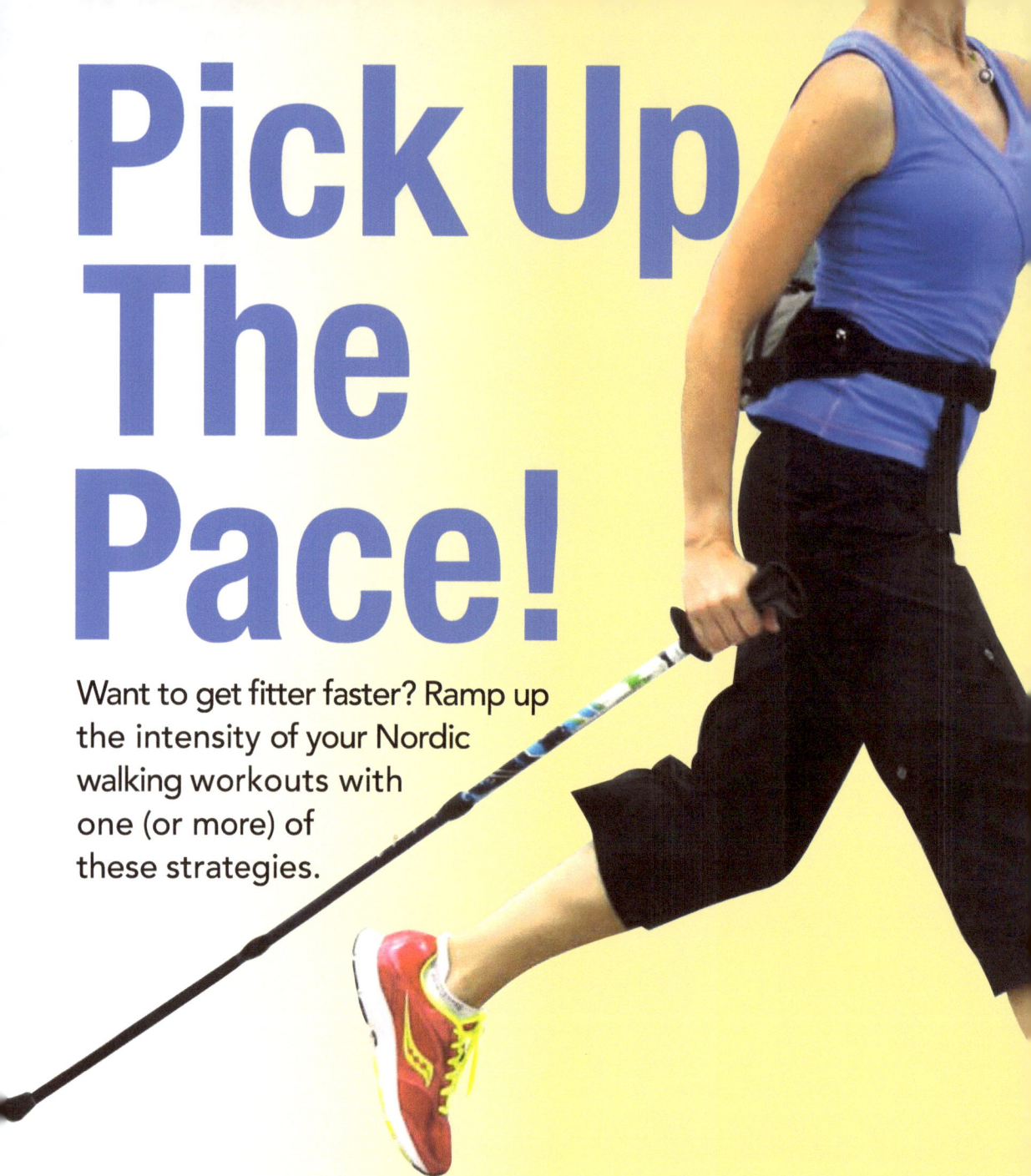

1 DOUBLE-CHECK YOUR FORM

Is your technique as perfect as possible? Have a friend videotape you in action to see for yourself. If you exercise in a group, offer helpful critiques of each other's style. (And check back to page 12 if you need a technique refresher.)

2 HIT THE ACCELERATOR

To increase your speed, don't simply move your feet faster. Instead, press harder onto the Ledge of your handles. This will make your arms move faster (and work harder), which will require your legs to move faster to keep in sync.

3 FIND A FAST FRIEND

Make a date with a more-experienced Nordic walker to soak up his or her polished technique and to experience a faster-paced workout.

4 ADD STAIRS AND HILLS

Start with one flight or one hill, and build up to more as you're able. Use your poles to propel you to the top. On stairs move quickly, but play it safe by holding the railing with one hand and carrying your poles in the other.

5 MIX IT UP

Add intervals of high-intensity exercises, such as walking lunges, alternating high knee lifts or running.

6 THINK ARMS NOT LEGS

Try to make each step the result of pressing on the Ledge of your handles. Consciously work to make your legs less dominant.

7 INITIATE FROM THE SHOULDERS

While the push onto the Ledge of your handles is ultimately what propels you forward, try initiating the pushing action from your shoulders: Swing your arm forward, press your shoulder down, and feel that energy move down your arm and onto the Ledge.

8 STREAMLINE YOUR BODY

Don't waste energy swinging your arms even slightly away from the sides of your thighs. Instead, keep your arms and poles close to your body. Feel your hands regularly brush the sides of your thighs.

9 THINK HORIZONTAL

Avoid a bouncy up and down action as you walk. Instead, as you press your arms down and back, feel your body surge forward between your poles in a strong horizontal line.

10 LOOSEN YOUR SHOULDERS

Be sure you aren't tensing your shoulders in an effort to move faster. Instead, keep your shoulders (and your grip) very loose so your arms swing forward and backward very freely. Consciously work to make your legs less dominant.

Get Out
of Town

Hiking, bushwalking, tramping or trekking. Whatever you call it, step out of your comfort zone and take your poles on an adventure. Follow these 14 tips for using your poles on adventurous terrain.

1. On trails and grass, **remove your boot tips**. Let the carbide tips of your poles dig into the soft surface.

2. **Add trekking baskets** to keep your poles from sinking between large rocks or into very muddy soil.

3. On staircases, long or steep hills, and when your footing is unsure, temporarily **forego your Nordic walking technique**; instead, utilize any technique that helps you balance and stabilize your body. For example, you may want to bend your elbows and plant your boot tips beside or in front of your feet. Once the surface levels out and smoothes out, transition back into Nordic walking technique.

4. **Shorten your poles** for an extended uphill climb; lengthen your poles for an extended downhill climb.

5. To avoid grip fatigue on long outings, **consider changing your hand position** occasionally by placing your hands on the Palm (the top) of the handles.

6. On adventure holidays, Urban Poling's Adventure poles are the best option because they telescope down to a small size that fits into most suitcases. When they aren't being used, you can easily **store them in your backpack**.

7. **Don't leave your poles lying outside** on the ground overnight. Small rodents are sometimes attracted to the salty sweat on the handles, and they may chew them.

8. When travelling by airplane, **pack your poles in your checked luggage**, not in your carry-on luggage. Or use your poles to walk through security, stating that they are a mobility aid if asked. Or consider taking a doctor's letter that states this, especially if you are younger and don't appear to require them as a walking aid. Airport security in some countries is stricter than others. Keep the boot tips on (in case the carbide tips appear weapon-like), and refer to them simply as walking poles.

9. When adventuring in a group, **stick an address label** or a piece of bright tape onto your poles so you can quickly identify them as yours.

10. **Wrap a long length of duct tape** around one of your poles. Use it to repair a damaged hiking boot or jacket or even to wrap a sprain.

11. Lightweight **high-cut hiking boots** with a soft upper material, paired with anti-blister socks, are a must for rocky surfaces and cobblestones. Lighter walking shoes are ideal for smoother terrain in cities and towns.

12. **Beware of ticks**, blood-feeding parasites that live in tall grass and can carry diseases such as Lyme disease. Ticks can latch onto shoes, socks or clothing and then work their way up your body until they find exposed skin. To avoid them, wear a hat, long-sleeved shirt, and long pants with the legs tucked into your socks. Use insect repellents with DEET, and learn how to do a post-walk "tick check." Wearing light coloured clothing makes them easier to spot.

13. **When packing your poles** in a suitcase, make them as short as possible by carefully pulling the two or three sections apart and removing the boot tips.

14. **Always travel with at least one extra pair** of boot tips. If you lose one or both, they may be difficult to replace in a foreign country. 🏃

Nordic Walking HIIT* Workout

high intensity interval training

Warm up, and then perform as many repetitions as possible each of the following exercises for 20 seconds. Rest for 10 seconds between exercises. Repeat the circuit 1–3 times. Modify the exercises as required.

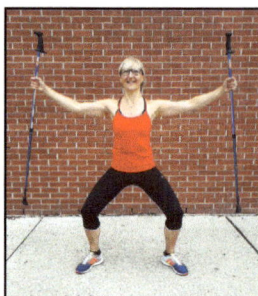
jumping jacks

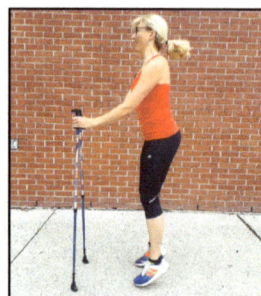
squat jumps

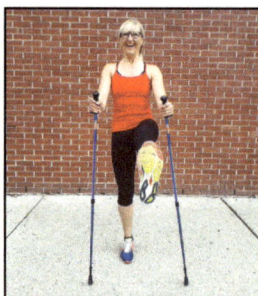
front kicks

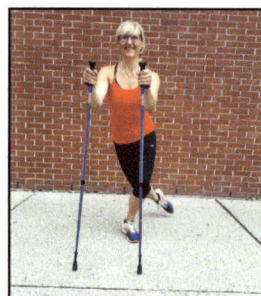
skater hops

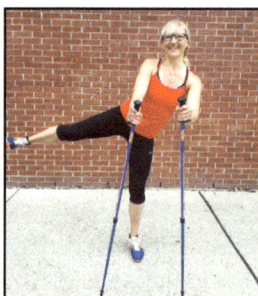
side kicks

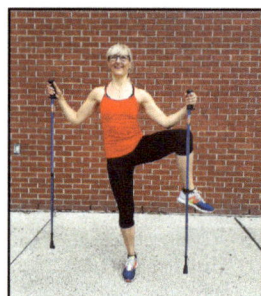
Spiderman knee lifts

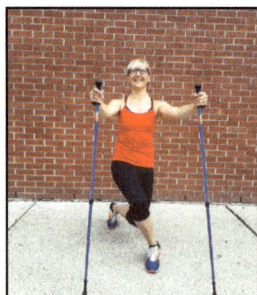
curtsey lunges

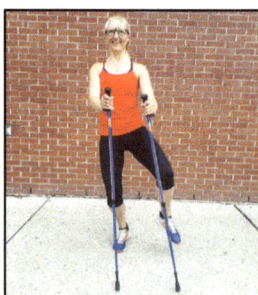
football run

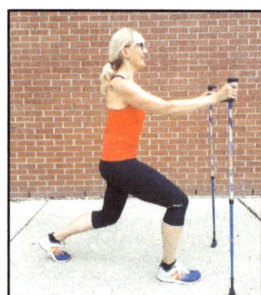
jumping lunges

Pilates on the Move

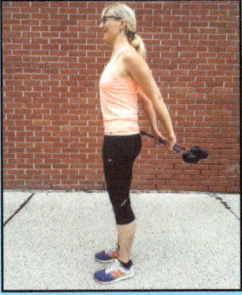
triceps pressbacks

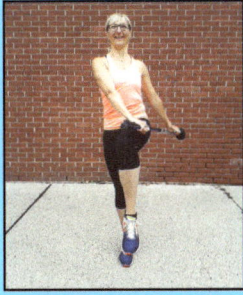
crisscross knee lifts

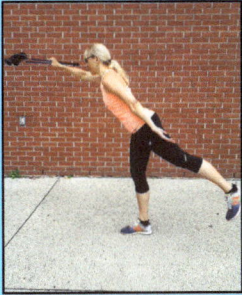
bird dogs

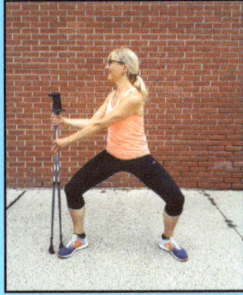
spinal twist & plant

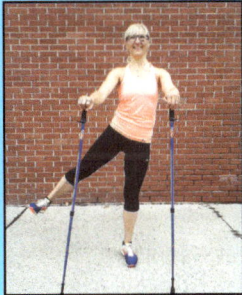
side leg lifts

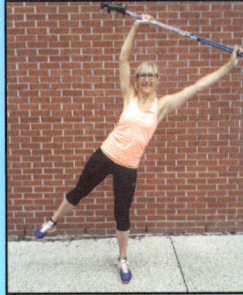
overhead reaches

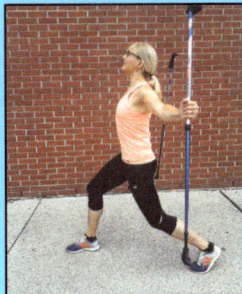
lunges

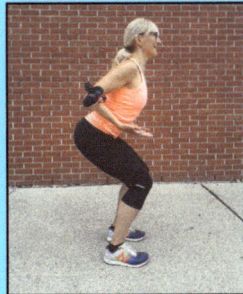
squats

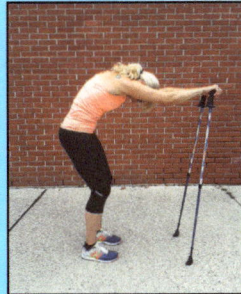
cat stretch

Pilates and Nordic walking both focus strongly on core conditioning and precise movement technique. This Pilates-inspired workout is ideal for anyone seeking improved all-over fitness, including cyclists, dragon boaters and golfers. Perform one minute of each exercise, resting for 5-10 seconds between exercises. Repeat the sequence twice.

The Joy of Snowshoeing

One of world's oldest sports gets a boost by adding poles

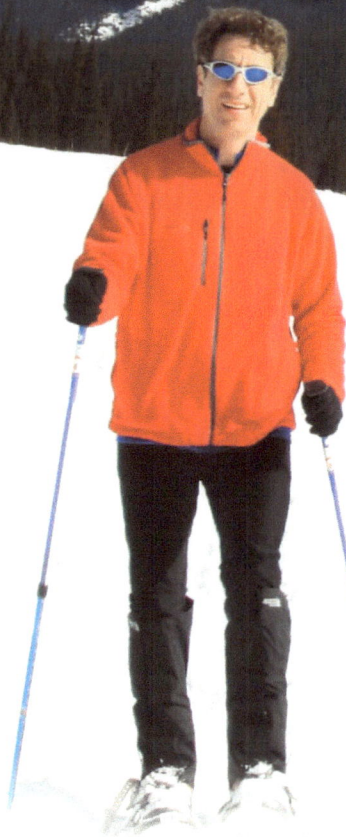

WEIGH THE OPTIONS

Choose the right style of snowshoes: recreational (for first-timers and simple terrain); fitness (a more-rugged design and ideal for running); and backpacking (extremely strong and for powder snow).

RENT OR BUY

You can rent snowshoes for $15–$20 per day from an outdoors store or ski resort. Or pay $150–$200 for an entry-level pair with good quality bindings, which will release easily at the end of your walk even if they're covered in ice and snow.

ADD SNOW BASKETS

Attach snow baskets to the end of your poles. They will keep the tips of your poles up on top of the snow, preventing them from sinking and disappearing.

FOLLOW THE RULES

Any park, field or trail with fresh snow is perfect for snowshoeing. Many resorts have cross country ski trails that snowshoers can share. Just follow trail etiquette and walk beside, not on, the cross country ski tracks.

"Snowshoeing with poles is a fabulous workout," says Urban Poling certified instructor Lois Tomlinson, who leads snowshoe outings through her Vancouver company, Natural Trekking Tours. "Snowshoes weigh about two pounds each, so walking in fresh snow and up and down hills can really get your heart pumping. And adding poles with snow baskets helps you balance on tricky terrain, challenges your upper body muscles and zaps more calories."

FLEX YOUR TECHNIQUE

Standard Nordic walking technique works well on snowy, flat and wide trails and fields. But on hills, narrow trails and rough footing, stabilize yourself by bending your elbows and using your poles hiking-style.

DRESS FOR SUCCESS

Wear snow-repellant ski clothes, not jeans, since some snowshoes kick up a rooster tail of snow behind you. Sunscreen and sunglasses are also a must to protect you from the blinding sun reflecting off the snow.

THINK DRINK

It is as important to drink fluids during cold weather as it is in hot weather. Use an insulated water bottle to keep your water from freezing. Or carry a hot drink in a thermos, which will keep you hydrated, nourished and warm.

PRACTISE FALLING

If you will be walking on challenging terrain, practise recovering from a fall. To get up, roll onto your side, tuck your knees under you, and then use your poles to help you stand.

WATCH YOUR STEP

A good pair of snowshoes requires little or no maintenance. They'll last for years as long as you don't damage the crampons (the metal teeth on the bottom) by walking on gravel or pavement.

NORDIC WALKING ADVENTURES

Conquered your neighbourhood sidewalks and parks?
Consider one of these walking events, fundraisers or adventurous routes.

1. **Terry Fox Run/Walk** (*www.terryfox.org*): a non-competitive cancer fundraiser held in 25+ countries

2. **Oxfam Trailwalker** (*www.oxfamtrailwalker.org*): 2-day, 200 km/125 mile team event held in 11 countries

3. **The Camino de Santiago** (*thecamino.com.au*): 800 km/500 mile route starting in France and finishing in Spain

4. **Great Walks of New Zealand** (*www.newzealand.com*): multi-day walks that journey through the country's most magnificent landscapes and iconic locations

5. **The Coast to Coast Walk** (*www.coast2coast.co.uk*): 309 km/192 mile unofficial and mostly unsignposted footpath in Northern England that passes through three national parks

6. **Arthritis walking events**: *www.arthritis.ca; www.arthritisaustralia.com; www.arthritis.org*

7. **Diabetes walking events**: *www.diabetes.ca; www.diabetesaustralia.com.au ; www.diabetes.org; www.diabetes.org.uk*

8. **Breast cancer walking events**: *www.cbcf.org; www.avon39.org; www.cancer.org; www.breastcanceruk.org.uk; www.bcna.org.au.*

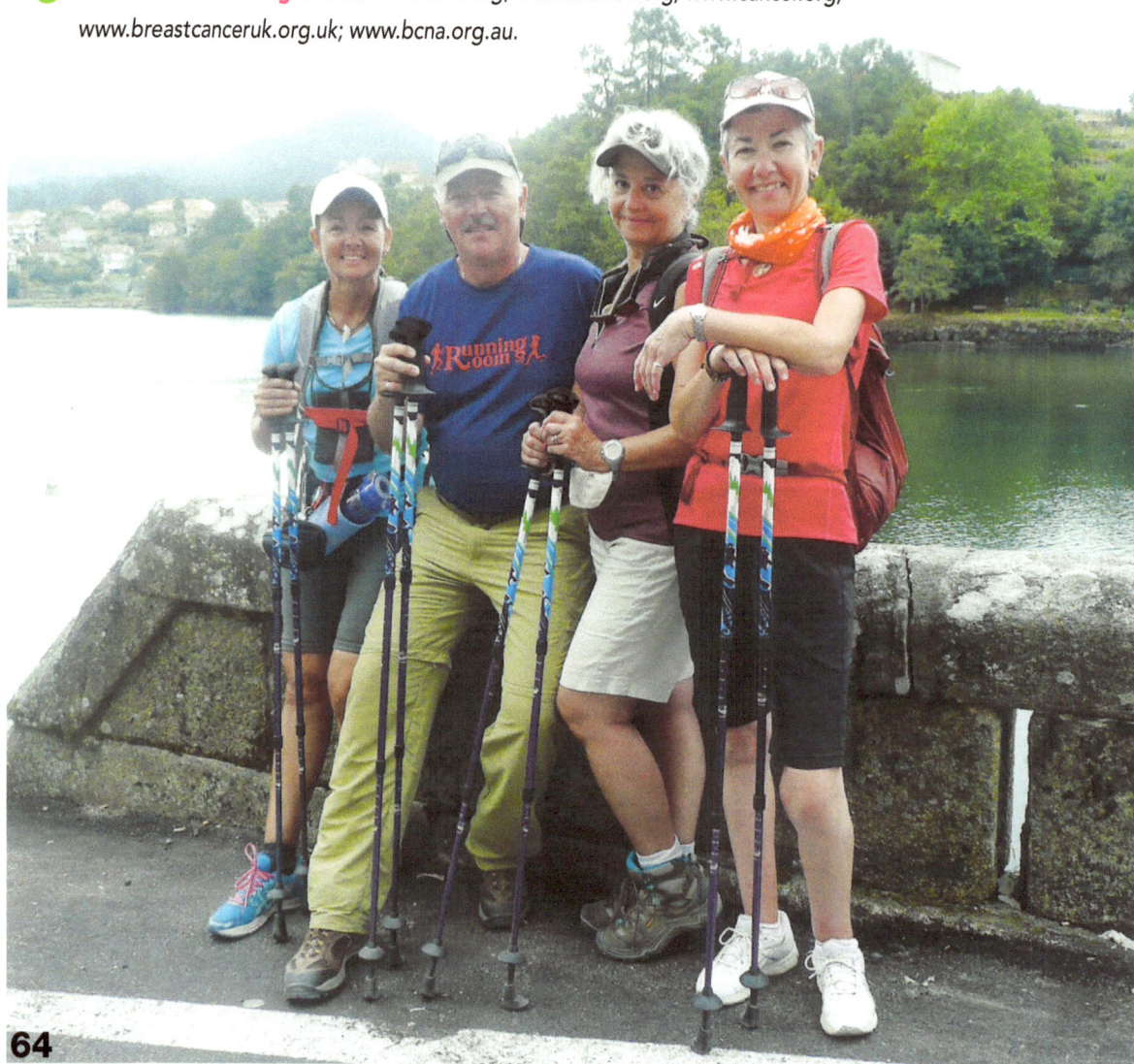

URBANPOLING

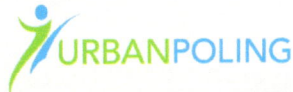

Beginner's Checklist to Nordic Walking Success

☐ Purchase high quality Nordic walking poles (visit www.urbanpoling.com to find a retailer or to order online).

☐ Get the right clothing (see page 16).

☐ Set up your poles correctly (see page 10).

☐ Learn the technique (see page 12), or visit www.urbanpoling.com for online tips and the "Find a Class" tab to register for a clinic or series of classes in your town or city.

☐ Set a benchmark and then track your progress (see "How Fit Are You?" on page 18).

☐ Use your poles regularly so the technique eventually feels natural.

☐ Introduce your partner, family and friends to Nordic walking (research shows that adding a social aspect to exercise greatly increases adherence).

☐ Follow Urban Poling on Facebook and Twitter to share your successes, tips and photos, or connect via email (barb@urbanpoling.com).

Get to Know Your ACTIVATOR® Walking Poles

Which Poles are Best for Me?

Choose the **ACTIVATOR** walking poles if you answer YES to any of these statements:

1. I feel unsteady or somewhat unsteady on my feet when walking..
   YES ☐ NO ☐

2. I currently walk with a cane.
   YES ☐ NO ☐

3. My health care professional suggested that the **ACTIVATOR** poles may help me be more active and walk with more confidence.
   YES ☐ NO ☐

Choose the **ACTIVATOR²** walking poles if you *also* answer YES to either of these statements:

1. I am taller than six feet/183 cm.
   YES ☐ NO ☐

2. I want poles that compress to fit into a suitcase.
   YES ☐ NO ☐

The ACTIVATORS may be ideal for people with these health conditions (and with your health care professional's approval): hip and knee issues (before surgery and after post-surgery therapy), soft tissue injuries (after acute phase), osteoporosis, mild stroke, acquired brain injury, spinal stenosis (after surgery), cardiac issues, arthritis (except severe rheumatoid arthritis affecting hand strength), early stages of Parkinson's and multiple sclerosis (not for ataxia), respiratory conditions (after acute phase and once stable) and breast cancer (after acute phase of surgery/treatment).

CoreGrip handle, Ledge,   **upper section**   **lower section**   **bell shape tip**

silver button

velcro wrap

Set Up Your ACTIVATOR Poles

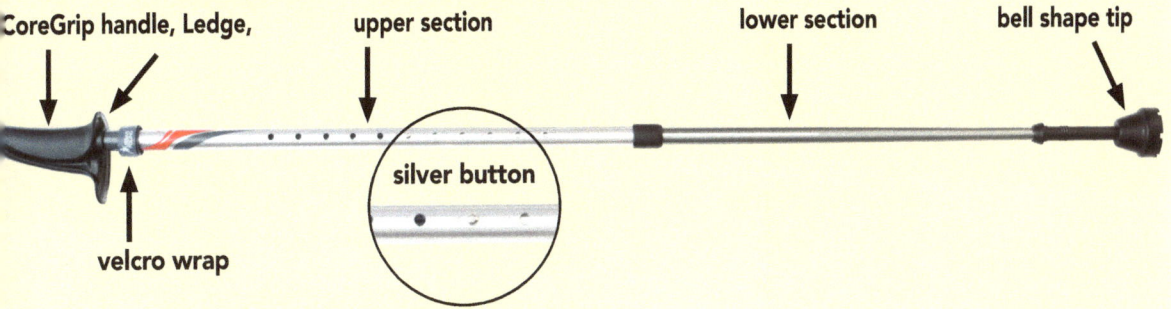

1. Pull out the lower section until you see a white stripe running the length of it (you may need to twist the lower section to find the stripe).

2. Align the stripe with the perforated holes of the upper section. Slide the lower section up and down until a silver button pops into any hole.

3. When you stand holding the handles with your elbows at your sides and the poles vertical, your elbows should be slightly below a 90° angle. Use the button to lengthen or shorten your poles.

4. Hold the Right and Left poles in the appropriate hands.

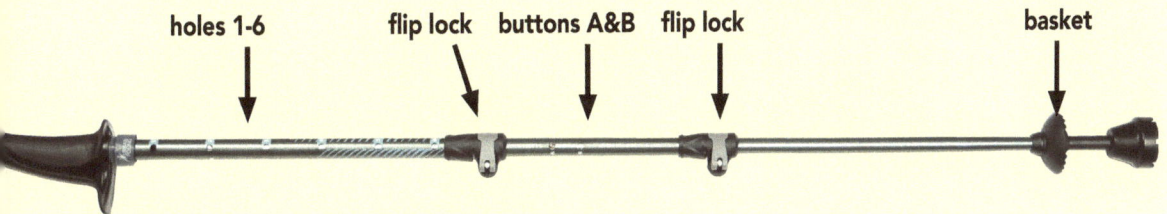

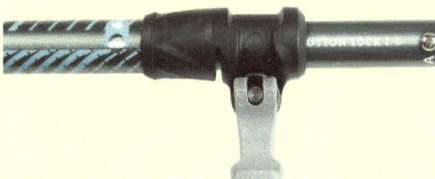

holes 1-6   **flip lock**   **buttons A&B**   **flip lock**   **basket**

Set Up Your ACTIVATOR^2 Poles

1. Open both flip-locks. Extend the middle section and lower section of the pole. When you stand holding the handles with your elbows at your sides and the poles vertical, your elbows should be slightly below a 90° angle.

2. Turn the lower section until a white stripe appears in holes A and B. Adjust the lower section until a button pops into hole A or B.

3. Repeat Step 2 with the upper section, securing a second button in a hole marked 1-6. Confirm that the pole length is correct, and close the flip locks.

4. Hold the Right and Left poles in the appropriate hands.

67

How to Walk With Your ACTIVATOR® Poles

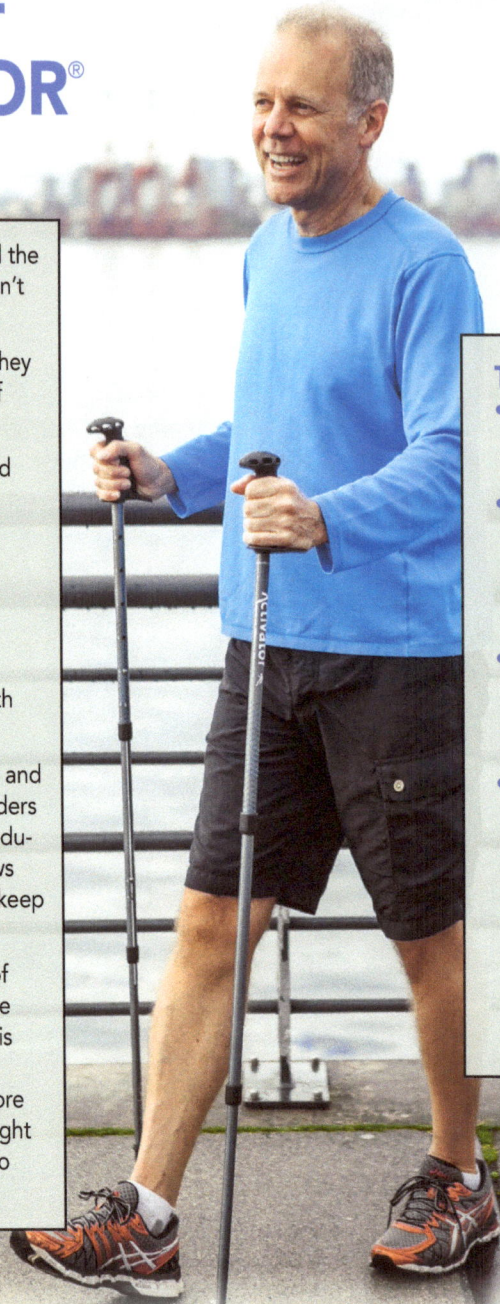

1. **Wrap** your fingers around the CoreGrip handles, but don't squeeze them too tightly.

2. **Plant** your poles so that they are vertical and in front of your feet at all times.

3. **Coordinate** your arms and legs as with standard walking: move your right leg and left arm forward simultaneously, then your left leg and right arm.

4. **Plant** the bell shape tip beside your front foot with each step.

5. **Swing** your arms forward and backward from the shoulders (not the elbows), like pendulums, keeping your elbows bent at all times. Do not keep your upper arms static.

6. **Press** the outside edge of your hands firmly onto the Ledge of the handles. This increases your stability, activates your arm and core muscles and offloads weight from your lower body into the poles.

TIPS

- **DO** stand as tall as possible with your shoulders over your hips and your navel pulled up and in.
- **DO** start walking quite slowly, even somewhat robotically. Once the action begins to feel natural, move more smoothly and perhaps a little faster.
- **DO**, as an option, remove the bell shape tip to make use of the basket when walking on sand and soil.
- **DO** progress to Nordic walking poles (and Nordic walking technique) if your health care provider recommends this. Replace your ACTIVATOR poles with Nordic walking poles, or replace your ACTIVATOR's bell shape tips with Nordic walking boot shape tips.

IMPORTANT

- For more information, read the ACTIVATOR User's Guide, and watch the ACTIVATORS in action at www.urbanpoling.com.
- Direct your health care professional to www.urbanpoling.com for training courses, research information and webinars.
- If you use a cane, crutches or a walker, live with a medical condition that affects your balance, stability, hand strength, vision, depth perception or coordination, or are recovering from an injury or surgery, consult your health care professional before using the ACTIVATOR poles. People using two canes or a walker must use the ACTIVATOR poles under the supervision of a health care professional.

The Journey of the ACTIVATOR® Walking Poles

Every week I receive comments from people who have benefited tremendously from using our company's ACTIVATOR walking poles. This is extremely gratifying for me because it was a long and challenging journey to bring the ACTIVATORS to market.

Let me take you back many years to how it started.

Several years ago, when I was completing my Master's degree in gerontology, I had an interesting conversation with my Swedish neighbour who told me about the incredible popularity of Nordic walking in Scandinavia. As an occupational therapist, the many health benefits of the activity sparked my interest in the possibility of using walking poles for therapy purposes.

I was so intrigued by our conversation that I spent the following year evaluating the effectiveness of walking poles. I was excited to discover more than 50 research studies (today there are more than 100) showing that walking with poles may improve posture, balance and gait speed, reduce impact to the knees, provide good general physical conditioning, burn more calories than standard walking, strengthen the core muscles, and help people adhere to a regular walking regime.

This information led me to believe that walking poles might be a solution to a therapist's greatest frustration: clients who don't exercise consistently.

I co-founded Urban Poling Inc. in 2005 to develop a modified Nordic walking pole for adults and youth with disabilities, inactive older adults, and adults with mid- to later-stages of chronic health conditions, including arthritis, osteoporosis, Parkinson's disease, hip and knee replacements, and cardiac and cerebrovascular disease.

But just as we were launching, Nordic walking began to emerge in North America as a popular fitness activity. This led to a change in direction for the business. Instead of developing a rehab pole, we quickly changed gears and introduced a Nordic walking pole and a national training centre, which has to date trained over 5,000 instructors. The great success of our Nordic walking poles initially kept the company afloat so we could continue to work on what would become the ACTIVATOR rehabilitation poles.

Over many months, we developed more than 10 ACTIVATOR prototypes, using feedback from therapists and a university research study. Once the poles were designed, we developed an ACTIVATOR walking technique and a three-hour training program for therapists.

While the development process was incredibly challenging, it has been equally rewarding. I believe that the ACTIVATOR poles are revolutionizing the way that many therapists provide gait retraining and rehabilitation for their clients.

by Mandy Shintani, occupational therapist and co-director of Urban Poling Inc.

> **When my physician told me to use a cane, the word 'disability' came to mind, and I was so discouraged. With the ACTIVATORS, my first thought was 'ability.**
>
> Letty Kurucz, knee replacement client

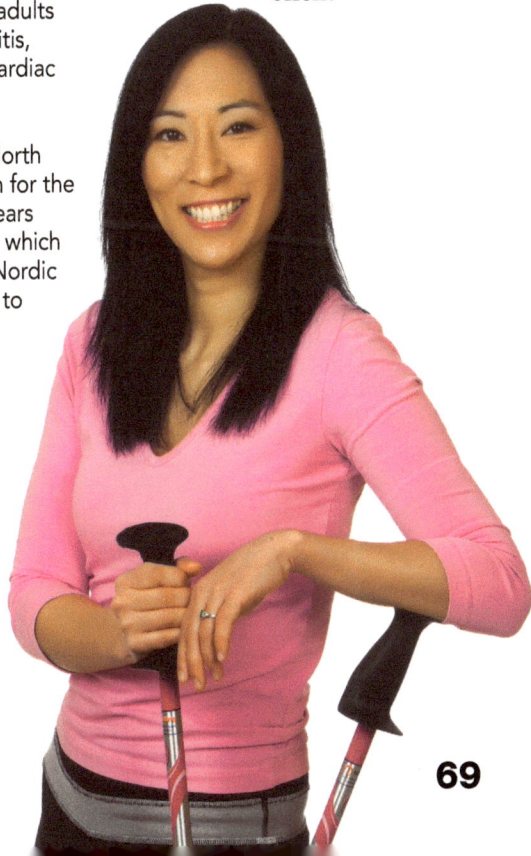

Seated ACTIVATOR® Exercises

Ask your health care provider to help you safely perform these exercises.

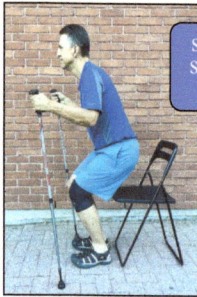
sit to stand

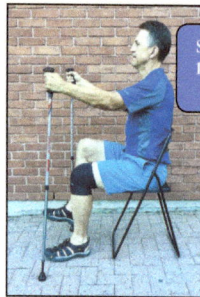
seated marching

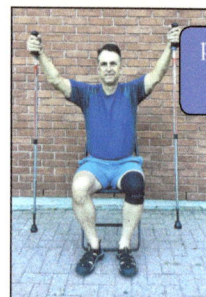
pole lifts

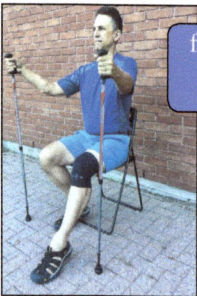
front taps

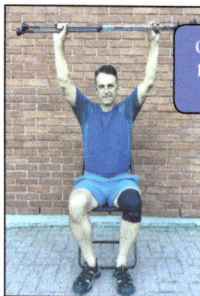
overhead reaches

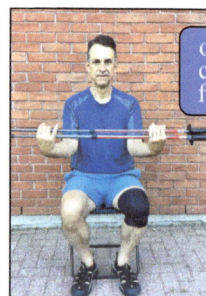
open & close fingers

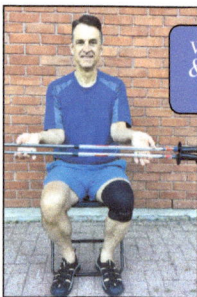
wrist flex & extend

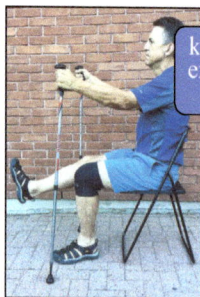
knee extensions

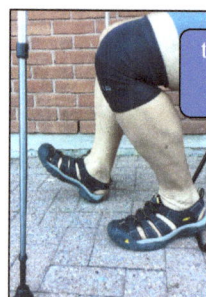
toe lifts

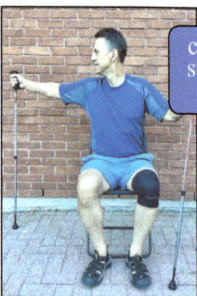
chest stretch

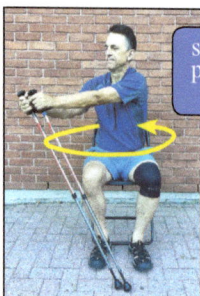
stir the pot

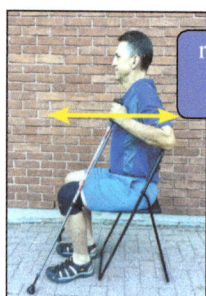
rows

Note: Use a sturdy chair, and place the back of it close to a wall.

Standing ACTIVATOR® Exercises

Ask your health care provider to help you safely perform these exercises.

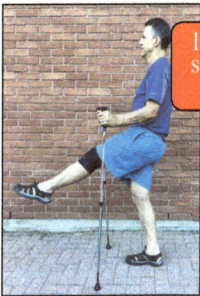
leg swings

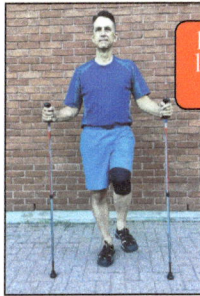
knee lifts

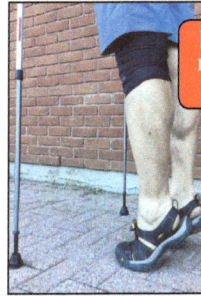
heel raises

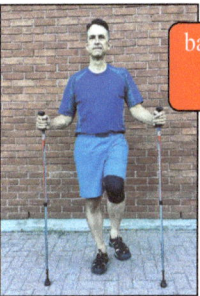
balancing

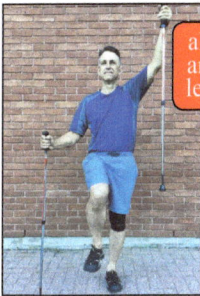
alternate arm & leg lifts

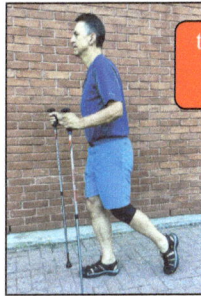
tap backs

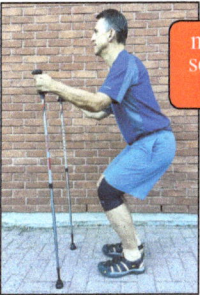
mini squats

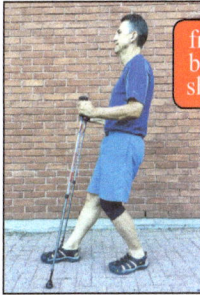
front & back weight shifting

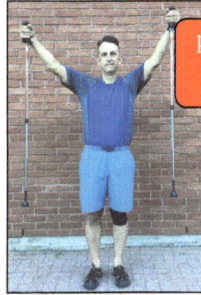
pole lifts

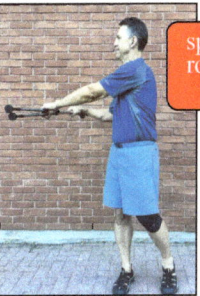
spine rotations*

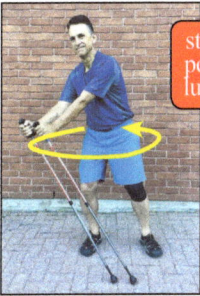
stir the pot & mini lunges*

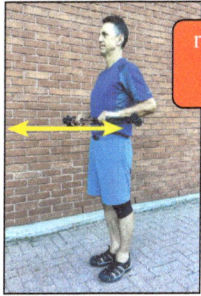
rows

*May not be suitable if you have back concerns.

It's a Wrap!

Congratulations—we've covered a lot of material here. Keep this book handy and refer to it often as you continue to build your Nordic walking skills and technique.

Can you handle just a bit more input? If that's a yes, here are a few final thoughts

Keep moving forward

The best way to become comfortable with your poles is to use them regularly. Enjoy energizing Nordic walks on your own, with a friend or in a group.

And don't be shy about getting out there. If you feel like a newbie today, just give it a couple of weeks. As soon as you meet someone just starting out with poles, you'll immediately feel like a seasoned pro.

Have fun

Every worthwhile goal takes time to achieve. Keep at it, and in just a few weeks you'll be glad you did.

Barb Gormley

Don't get stuck

Run into trouble? Still have questions?

Contact me at
Barb@urbanpoling.com
www.urbanpoling.com
www.BarbGormley.com

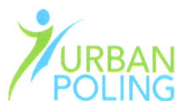

URBAN POLING

www.ingramcontent.com/pod-product-compliance
Lightning Source LLC
Chambersburg PA
CBHW060828270326
41931CB00003B/103